Why Diets Don't Work

Food Is Not the Problem

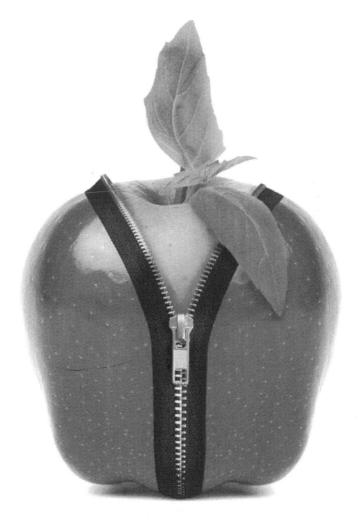

Joyce Tilney

Cover Design: Denise Rosser
Cover illustration©iStockphoto.com
Photograph: Sue Griffith

| ISBN13 | 978-0-615-61634-6 |
| ISBN-10: | 0615616348 |

Published by
The Voice of Grace and Truth
PO Box 43
Brandamore, PA 19316

Why Diets Don't Work: Food Is Not The Problem

Dedication

To my best friend and husband, Bill, who has been on this
journey with me every pound of the way!

Jeni Tilney Allen, my daughter, who has encouraged me throughout the
journey. Thanks for your input.

Bill Tilney, Jr., my son, who had confidence in me that I could conquer the
tech world and reach beyond myself to become part of the social media age.
Thanks for your help and encouragement.

Acknowledgement

Joyce Macias, Lindsay Tilney, Cindy Grant and Delia Diaz for all your help in editing, proofing and input. I appreciate your willingness to help.

Table of Contents

FORWARD IX

ENDORSEMENTS XI

INTRODUCTION XIII

1. HE SPOKE AND I WAS STRENGTHENED 1

2. A LACK OF PERCEPTION LEADS TO DECEPTION! 5

3. IT'S AN INSIDE JOB! 13

4. CREATED IN HIS IMAGE 21

5. THE BATTLE OF THE BULGE 33

6. YOU'VE BEEN AROUND THIS MOUNTAIN LONG ENOUGH!............41

7. FASTING: THE WEAPON OF CHOICE 49

8. NOTHING TASTES AS GOOD AS OBEDIENCE 59

9. IDENTITY: THE SECRET OF SUCCESS 67

10. DILIGENCE OVERCOMES DESPERATION!............................73

11. ONE MORE WORD 81

THE BATTLE PLAN 87

POINTS TO PONDER 91

ABOVE ALL ELSE 97

WORDS FOR THE WALK 99

SPIRIT FOOD FOR THE SPIRIT MAN......................................103

SOUL FOOD FOR THE SOUL 107

HEALTH FOOD FOR THE BODY..109

RECOMMENDED READING 111

ABOUT THE AUTHOR 115

WOMEN OF GOD MINISTRIES...117

SCHEDULE A "WHY WEIGHT" SEMINAR 123

Forward

As we go through this journey we call life we come across people that I consider divine appointments. Joyce Tilney was one of those divine appointments in my life. I first met her as she came to my publishing company and was seeking advice for writing several books that were in her heart to publish.

We were friends right then and there. Joyce is a woman of incredible character, strength, and great wisdom, but like many of us she struggled with a weight problem. Like Joyce, I too had weight issues as I got older, and I began to hold back in the ministry call on my life. I hadn't seen Joyce in a great while and one day she showed up at my door. We got caught up on all of the lost time and then she told me of a new book she had written, *Why Diets Don't Work*.

Now, here is a book you simply must read! As I read, the realization of where I was at with my weight issues became so clear and I became focused. I felt the victory finally for the first time in my life and I hadn't done anything but read! I knew from this book, *Why Diets Don't Work*, how to get the victory that had eluded me all these years. From the first chapter where she states, "The Devil wants you fat!" my eyes were open, my heart was ready, and my body was about to be changed into a healthy temple for God.

The message in this book can heal the emotional scars, the broken hearts and the weight issues of your life. She reveals the power of the

Holy Spirit to focus you on God's Word with "revelation." She explains in the book how you are a "servant of your choices." She has so many wonderful thoughts and ideas that she shares freely that you find yourself sighing a breath of fresh air because you are understanding the cause, the defeat and the tremendous solutions to end the weight nightmare for the rest of your life. Joyce makes it clear it is not a contest about losing pounds; it is about a life journey learning to make right choices with the benefit of losing weight.

It is not often that a publisher and editor will give forwards to books, but I simply must with *Why Diets Don't Work*. It is an answer to what ails you. It is a winner not only in the weight battle, but in walking in the Spirit of God with great peace and victory in all areas of your life. Joyce has written a book we can all benefit from even if we don't have weight issues. She has written how to walk with the Lord in total victory in your life!

Susan K. Reidel
Logos to Rhema Publishing

Endorsements

I highly recommend this book to all believers who desire to walk in the spiritual and physical health that God has destined for us.

This book is not a politically correct diet plan for those who want an easy way to lose weight; it is in fact a detailed strategy guide to combat the devil's intentions, meant to keep us from fulfilling God's design for our lives.

This is an inspirational book filled with daily health food for your spirit and soul. Come and dine!

Alta Hatcher
Director of Healing Ministries
Christ For The Nations

I've known Joyce many years. She's been a real encouragement to me both in ministry and personally. It never ceases to amaze me at the insight and revelation of God's Word which is consistently released into her life by the Holy Spirit of God. She hears and understands the voice of the Lord and the timing of releasing the revelation into the lives of others.

"Why Diet's Don't Work" is yet another valuable tool and revelation we all need to understand about dieting. Overeating does not start with food, but understanding our inner need for food and how the enemy works overtime in trying to keep us from seeing the truth of its origin.

Thank you Joyce for releasing the revelation you have received to those who struggle with their weight, including myself. Now is the time and season to allow the Lord to use this book and its revelation to break the chains which keep us from overcoming in this area of our lives.

Linda Patton

Seedtime & Harvest
London, England

Introduction

*"Unzipping" the truths of God's Word
to get to the core of the matter,
exposing the lies of the enemy!*

This is not another diet plan, it is a battle plan!

"The devil wants you fat!" When I read those words it was like an explosion in my spirit. It was a light bulb moment that completely changed my thinking about the fight I had been waging for years. I had always known the devil used my fat, but I had not thought about the fact that the devil actually wanted me fat. I immediately recalled the scripture, "the thief does not come except to steal, and to kill, and to destroy. I have come that they may have life and that they may have it more abundantly" (John 10:10 NKJV).

That's what this battle has been all about. The devil has been trying to wipe me out through obesity that opens the door for him to steal, kill and destroy. Obesity puts people at a greater risk for life-threatening illness like diabetes, heart disease and high blood pressure. Weight related problems have overtaken smoking and are now the single most preventable cause of illness and death in the United States. It is a source of poor self-image, depression and condemnation—all of which rob us of the gifts and talents that God has given us for His purposes.

How can this be? The 'diet' industry is a multi-million dollar business that is flourishing. There is a new diet with another magical cure every day, and yet we get fatter and fatter.

As Christians we have a tendency to classify sins. We look at the addiction to drugs, over-consumption of alcohol and pornography as sin, but we fail to grasp that the Bible has something to say about gluttony as well. Ezekiel 16:49 lists Sodom's sins as "pride, gluttony and laziness" (NLT). All overconsumption in any form goes against Christian teaching. We have become a nation of over-consumers!

Food is necessary for our survival. The devil used food when he tempted Eve. It worked so well, why should we be surprised when he continues to get us to take one more bite until we are in bondage to the taste, not the need for food?

After I saw the 'light' I began to seek the Lord diligently, asking Him to show me how to break the bondage that had become a disparaging part of my life. Throughout my life I have tried all the diets, been to all the programs and wasted thousands of dollars in the process. Of course, there was the wardrobe with four sizes as I went up and down the scale. Just like Eve, I thought a new dress would hide the sin.

Since becoming "born again" I always had a deep desire to overcome this battle God's way, but I couldn't see the way. The "light bulb" hadn't been turned on! Until we perceive things with our spiritual eyes and our understanding is enlightened, we will continue doing things the way the world does. "Do not be conformed to the world, but be transformed by the renewing of your mind, that you may prove what is that good and acceptable and perfect will of God" (Romans 12:2).

Introduction

When we are born again, conversion takes place in a moment but the transformation of the mind is an ongoing process as we grow in our ability to see and understand the ways of the Kingdom of Heaven. In order to change our lifestyle and daily choices, we must change the way we think.

To overcome any battle in life, we must understand ourselves and how we are created to function in this world as children of God. We must understand that God is a spirit, the devil is a spirit, and we have a spirit. We cannot fight this battle the world's way. "For we do not wrestle against flesh and blood, but against principalities, against powers, against the rulers of the darkness of this age, against spiritual hosts of wickedness in the heavenly places" (Ephesians 6:12). That is why we go up and down the scale. The devil has deceived us just like he did Eve. Until we understand this is a spiritual problem, we will continue on the roller coaster, endlessly fighting the battle of the bulge.

I know there are medical conditions that cause obesity. If this is your situation, please don't feel condemned. As I said before, this book is not a diet plan, but a battle plan. It addresses the spiritual issues that keep us from walking in obedience. Please check with your physician before going on any kind of diet or exercise program.

Eating is a necessary part of our lives; we do it every day and we need to treat our bodies well. It is the only one we have, and it is a gift from God. Everyone eats, but our motives are different. Some people want to gain weight, others want to lose weight. Whatever your desire is, we must learn to depend on the Holy Spirit to help us in our time of need.

As you read this book, I pray that the Holy Spirit unzips the truth to you and gives you a 'light-bulb' moment and you will walk in the freedom that God has provided for you through Jesus Christ. As children of God, we should be the happiest people on earth! We are on our way to heaven and God has provided everything we need to be happy on this earth!

Remember, you are not alone. You have a Helper, the Holy Spirit. Speaking to His disciples before leaving them, Jesus said in John 16:7, "Nevertheless I tell you the truth, it is to your advantage that I go away: for if I do not go away, the Helper will not come to you; but if I depart, I will send Him to you." You, as a child of God, have an advantage over the world! All you have to do is ask!"

 You are the apple of His eye

1

He Spoke and I Was Strengthened

"...So when He spoke to me I was strengthened and said, 'Let my lord speak, for you have strengthened me.'"

(DANIEL 10:19)

I will never forget the day I read John 10:4. "When He has brought out all His own, He goes on ahead of them, and His sheep follow Him because they know His voice" (NIV). They know His voice! As a new believer, I was so excited to think that I could hear God's voice. That He would speak to me personally. My faith was sparked. I expected to hear His voice! As I grew in my walk with the Lord and studied His word I understood there were different ways for Him to speak and direct us in our daily lives. He speaks to us through His Word, as we read it; He quickens our spirit by the Holy Spirit; His Spirit illuminates His word; He speaks through His servants, anointed pastors and teachers, and those who operate in the gifts of the Spirit - the word of wisdom and the word of knowledge. If you don't

1

understand about hearing the voice of the Lord, please study the Word of God regarding this. There are many good books that cover this subject in detail. But there is nothing like hearing that still small voice in your spirit, "and after the earthquake a fire, but the Lord was not in the fire; and after the fire a still small voice" (1 Kings 19:12).

So as I began my Christian walk I listened for that still small voice to lead me down the runway of life. Like everyone else I faced many struggles along the way.

The struggle with my weight started early in my life. I remember my first 'diet.' I was 10 years old and my mother took me to the doctor for tests. I became very conscious of my weight and learned to cover the hurt and abuse of others. During my high school years I managed to keep control of my weight although it was a constant battle. I married and had children and kept adding a little extra weight with each one.

I had been raised in a Christian home, but had turned away from God as a teenager. Nevertheless the seed of God's Word had been hidden in my heart from my Sunday school days. I knew something was missing in my life. Eventually my mother's prayers caught me and I prayed for Jesus to come into my life. Six months later my husband did the same thing and everything changed. Soon after we gave our lives to the Lord we found ourselves in Bible School preparing for ministry. The Lord blessed us as we moved to Scotland where we founded a church and I started a woman's ministry, Women of God, teaching women today from women of yesterday. As many ministers do, I got so busy that I didn't take care of myself as I should have. I was traveling to the nations, eating the wrong food at the wrong time and the weight began to slip on.

After eleven years in Scotland and traveling through Europe and Asia, the Lord brought us back to the United States. What an adjustment. Reverse culture shock hit hard! It seemed like I had no one to turn to. No one understood how I felt. Depression set in and I felt overwhelmed with life. The next time I stood on the scales I couldn't believe my eyes. I had gained 75 pounds! Now I was consumed with guilt and condemnation. I was ashamed. Nevertheless the Lord continued to open doors of ministry and I knew that God loved me no matter what my size was. When you are being led by God, under His anointing, it doesn't matter if you are a size 2 or 32. But I was aware of all the health issues that stem from obesity and knew that I had to do something. So I jumped into dieting with both feet and got swallowed up by the diet industry in the process. One program told me how many points I could have and that I could spend them on any food that I wanted—until I'd used up my points for the day. When I got on the scales they loved me whether I lost weight or not and promised to love me as long as I came to their meeting and paid my dues. Another program delivered the perfect frozen dinners to my door with a promise of weight loss. Try as I might, each diet program left me feeling defeated and hopeless.

Lord, I cried, "There must be an answer to this problem". I made a decision that I would not try another diet plan. I knew that God had a solution and I began calling out for help! I don't recall how long it was after that decision, but one day I saw the words, "the devil wants you fat!" These words hit me like a ton of bricks! The devil used my fat against me all the time in making me feel guilty and ashamed leading to discouragement and depression. I knew that, but for some reason I had never thought about the fact that he wanted me fat.

Now that may sound silly to you, but it is the truth. I hate the devil. I had watched as he tried to destroy my family with drugs and alcohol. But it had just never occurred to me he was using food addiction to destroy me. The devil wanted me fat! These words just pierced my heart! Immediately, the Holy Spirit brought to my remembrance, "the thief does not come except to steal, and to kill, and to destroy. I have come that they may have life and that they may have it more abundantly" (John 10:10). I realized that this was an area of my life where the thief was stealing my joy and he was in the process of destroying my health. I certainly was not living an abundant life (except in fat cells). On top of that the enemy was stealing my finances as I bought new clothes to cover my sin just as Eve tried to cover her sin with a new garment of fig leaves.

So, I continued to cry out, "Lord, I need to hear from you. I need a word from you to cut asunder the thick cords of the wicked." One day during my devotion time, I heard that still small voice, "Break the habit." I knew exactly what He was talking about—my eating habit. Was it really that simple, as simple as breaking a habit? I soon found out that breaking a habit required facing a number of challenges. The devil was not about to give up without a fight. BUT, I had a word from God. I knew His voice and I knew exactly what He was saying. He spoke and I was strengthened.

"...and the sheep follow him, because
they know his voice."

(JOHN 10:4 NIV)

A Lack of Perception Leads to Deception!

"But I fear, lest somehow, as the serpent deceived Eve by his craftiness, so your minds may be corrupted from the simplicity that is in Christ."

(2 CORINTHIANS 11:3)

What really happened in the garden? Paul was concerned that our minds would be corrupted just like Eve. If ever a woman had everything going her way it was Eve! She was the first woman, first wife and first mother. She had it all. She was there 'in the beginning,' immediately after God created the world. Everything was beautiful. The air was fresh and the water was pure. All of creation lived in harmony. Her marriage seemed to be perfect and her relationship with God was a joy. God blessed them and told them to be fruitful and multiply. He provided them with everything they needed.

All He asked in exchange was that they leave one tree alone: "Of every tree of the garden you may freely eat; but of the tree of the knowledge of good and evil you shall not eat for in the day that you eat of it you shall surely die" (Genesis 2:16-17).

Although God had given Adam and Eve specific instructions not to eat of the tree, he had also given them a free will and the ability to make choices. They had a choice to make about this tree. God didn't want them eating its fruit because He did not want them to have the knowledge of evil. At this point all they knew was good. God Himself had called His creation "good" and "very good." God wanted to spare them from evil, just as He desires that for us today. What they learned, when they took fruit from the tree and ate, has been passed down through the entire human line, leaving us vulnerable to choosing evil instead of good, or even good instead of the best that God wants for us.

> The devil always points out the short-term benefit, never the long term effect.

Eve, the woman who had everything, was distracted by a voice. The devil brought her attention to the tree. There is no indication Eve had given any thought to the tree or had any curiosity about it until the devil asked his question, "Has God indeed said, "You shall not eat of every tree of the garden?" (Genesis 3:1).

Eve's response shows us her problem. "We may eat the fruit of the trees of the garden; but of the fruit of the tree which is in the midst of the garden, God has said, 'You shall not eat it, nor shall you touch it, lest you die'" (Genesis 3:2-3). God said nothing about touching the tree. Satan twisted God's Word and Eve added to it. This perversion of truth ultimately led to the fall of man.

Eve not only allowed the enemy to distract her, she engaged him in conversation. This always leads to trouble since he never has your best interest at heart. He doesn't mention the downside of disobedience. The devil always points out the short-term benefit, never the long-term effect. When he whispers enticements in our ear he leaves out important facts, like drinking alcohol can make a person an alcoholic, smoking cigarettes can cause lung cancer or eating too much of the wrong foods can lead to chronic illness and premature death. Instead, he emphasizes the aroma of the enticing dessert, the image that smoking is "cool" or the escape available in a glass of liquor.

Satan tempted Eve with the lust of the flesh, the lust of the eyes, and the pride of life (1John 2:16). Eve traded the eternal for the temporary, the truth for a lie. It looked good and she ate! Satan always baits deception with a little bit of truth. The devil's one trick worked so well on Eve that he is still using it today to turn our eyes from God's Word.

She had allowed the devil to distract her and let her mind think on the lies of the enemy. By doing this she lost her perfect communion with God even though she was still in the perfect place. She was no longer in a spiritual position to hear God's voice. She had given in to the temptation of the devil. Eating the fruit was evidence of what was in her heart. Eve did not perceive that she had been deceived!

When God approached Adam and Eve after their fall, He did not come with accusation, but with a question. "Where are you?" (Genesis 3: 9). He was not asking where they were physically, but about their position in the spirit. In that one question He was asking, "Where are you in your relationship with me? Where are you in the plans and purposes that I have for you?

God speaks to believers' spirits today just as He spoke to Adam and Eve in the garden. He has not changed. He is the same yesterday, today and forever. There is no room for argument or manipulating the voice of the Lord. God's Word was the standard in the garden, as it is now. It is the standard from which the actions of men and women must be judged as to whether they were right or wrong.

The devil's attack in the Garden was not against Eve, but against God's Word. Regardless of what he said, the devil did not care about Eve or her welfare. Just as God has not changed, neither has the devil. The enemy still comes to steal, kill and destroy. He is not creative, he is repeating the same attacks today as in the garden, trying to distract with one hand while deceiving us with the other.

He wants to distract us from the right path. He makes an enticing diversion from what is right and we become fascinated with something that is wrong. The mind is an open door for distraction for the person who has not hidden the Word of God in his or her heart. "Your word I have hidden in my heart that I might not sin against you" (Psalm 119:11).

The Genesis account doesn't say how many times Eve was tempted by the enemy, but the beginning of her downfall was when she listened to the enemy and pondered his words. She traded the security and strength that comes from God's Word for the temptation of the enemy. The enemy takes his time to set people up, one little thought at a time, and he does not give up easily.

Eve lost her position in the spirit where she could commune with God because she listened to and believed a lie of the enemy and gave in to his temptation. As a child of God we must protect our position in Christ so we can perceive when we are being deceived. Eve was still physically in the beautiful garden, but she was out of position in the spirit and was not sensitive and alert to the temptation of the enemy. Our position in the spirit gives us the authority over our enemy. "Behold, I give you the authority to trample on serpents and scorpions, and over all the power of the enemy, and nothing shall by any means hurt you" (Luke 10:19).

A Lack of Perception Leads to Deception!

Just like Eve, we can also allow distractions to cause us to lose our position in the spirit where we can hear His voice. We must continue to grow in the grace and knowledge of God and have fellowship through prayer and praise. Attending church every Sunday may put a person in the right place physically, but does not guarantee the ability to hear His voice. The fact that you live in the physical world does not determine your position in the spirit, but your spiritual position should affect your place in the natural world. The good news is we have been redeemed from the curse placed in the garden after the fall (Genesis 3:14-19). Galatians 3:13 says, "Christ has redeemed us from the curse of the law, having become a curse for us (for it is written, 'cursed is everyone who hangs on a tree')." Jesus went to the cross to restore the relationship with God that had been lost in the garden. He promised that He would never leave us or forsake us and that He would send a helper. "Nevertheless I tell you the truth, it is to your advantage that I go away; for if I do not go away, the Helper will not come to you; but if I depart, I will send Him to you" (John 16:7). Are you taking advantage of the helper that Jesus has given to you?

The role of the Holy Spirit is to help us face the temptation of the enemy by helping us recognize the devil's fingerprints all over the things that activate the cravings of our flesh, the enticement of our eyes and our personal ambitions. It's not so much that it's wrong to be hungry for a good meal or to enjoy looking at something pleasant or to have goals you are working toward. Again, the devil's tool is distraction, to get us so focused on the things of the world that we lose focus on our relationship with the Lord. Once he's drawn

> Jesus went to the cross to restore the relationship with God that had been lost in the garden.

our attention to things that are harmful for us, it's easy to make us feel deprived if we don't partake, like when we see other people eating whatever they want, when they want and never gain a pound! We forget that food is harming their body as it does ours, even if they are skinny!

> Our desire should not be to be a size 4, but to be healthy and happy as God created us to be.

Whether we are addicted to food, drugs or alcohol, God has made a way of escape. "Delight yourself also in the Lord, and He shall give you the desires of your heart" (Psalm 34:4). Our desire should not be to be a size 4, but to be healthy and happy as God created us to be. We cannot allow the world to form us into its image. Some of the most beautiful people I know could never make it in a beauty contest. Yet, their inner radiance, the life of Christ shining through them far surpasses any outer beauty! We are created in His image and His likeness. "For the Kingdom of God is not eating and drinking but righteousness and peace and joy in the Holy Spirit" (Romans 14:17). When you walk in a room people should know there is something different about you. Your spirit of joy and peace should shine forth and give beauty to your physical appearance.

We must heed Paul's warning and not allow our mind to be corrupted from the simplicity that is in Christ. When we allow the enemy to distract us in our mind we open the door to deception. Deception is being convinced that what is wrong is right. To perceive is to recognize, discern, envision or understand. A lack of perception leads to deception! What you perceive you believe. Only as our mind is renewed will we have the ability to guard our mind from the corruption of the enemy.

"There is therefore now no condemnation to those who are in Christ Jesus, who do not walk according to the flesh, but according to the Spirit."

(ROMANS 8:1)

3

It's an Inside Job!

---

*"…work out your own salvation with fear and trembling;
for it's God who works in you both to will and to do for His
good pleasure."*

(PHILIPPIANS 2:12-13)

As a child of God one of the first things we must understand is what happened when we were born again. We look the same, we think the same—so what happened? "For as in Adam all die, even so in Christ all shall be made alive" (1Corinthian 15:22). Adam and Eve lost fellowship with God because they were disobedient. God had told them, "…for in the day that you eat of it you shall surely die" (Genesis 2:17). They did not die a physical death, but a spiritual death; they were separated from God, they could no longer communicate with Him.

The good news is what was lost in the Garden of Eden was restored in the Garden of Gethsemane! When you are born again it is a spiritual birth restoring your communication with God. You are

13

now a child of God. "He came to His own, and His own did not receive Him. But as many as received Him to them He gave the right to become children of God, to those who believe in His name" (John 1:11-12). You now have the ability to fellowship and communicate with God. What had been stolen in the garden by our enemy, the devil, has been restored by Jesus Christ.

It doesn't take too long to figure out that we have an enemy! The truth is, we always had an enemy but our conversion gives us the ability to understand who our enemy is and how to overcome him. John 3:3 says, "Most assuredly, I say to you, unless one is born again he cannot see the kingdom of God." We have been translated from the kingdom of darkness into the kingdom of light. Our spiritual eyes are opened and we see the deception and ways of the enemy.

> It doesn't take too long to figure out that we have an enemy!

When we are born again we begin our journey with God, our Father. We have our Basic Instruction Book, the Bible, and our helper, the Holy Spirit to teach us. Romans 12:2 gives us specific instructions for life as a child of God. "And do not be conformed to this world, but be transformed by the renewing of your mind, that you may prove what is that good and acceptable and perfect will of God." We no longer need to depend on the world and its ways, if we choose to live God's ways by renewing our minds. We have to change our mind before we change our body, our life style and our health. The word 'transform' means to change markedly the form or appearance of, to change the nature, function or condition of, to convert. This only comes one way, by renewing our minds. Then we can see things from God's perspective. His ways and His thoughts are higher than ours (Isaiah. 55:9). He is always working in us for His good pleasure which is to perfect those things that concern us.

As a child of God we live from the inside out. We must become healthy on the inside before we are truly healthy on the outside. God works within us and we must work out our own salvation by living from the inside out! A simple truth is our brain has to change the way it thinks and we must learn patience in our body as the process takes place.

Our body reflects the daily choices that we make, so we must stop confusing our body by constantly changing our mind. Life is made up of choices and choices have consequences. Once we make a choice, we become the servant of that choice. "Do you not know that to whom you present yourselves slaves to obey, you are that one's slaves whom you obey, whether of sin leading to death, or of obedience leading to righteousness?" (Romans 6:16). Choices determine conduct and character. We alone are responsible for the choices we make. Poor food choices can become like a drug, sabotaging your body, draining your mental energy and making you feel hopeless. Choose your calories! Before you eat, think—is this food for fuel or fat? There is a power that is greater than our taste buds! A power that comes from the inside causing us to understand who we are and the power to live out that truth.

> Life is made up of choices and choices have consequences.

Food has always been an issue. It is not suddenly a new problem with an easy fix. We know that food was the enticement the devil used to cause Adam and Eve to sin in the Garden. They had been given authority over all things that God had created including the serpent.

> There is a power that is greater than our taste buds!

15

(Genesis 1:26) Why did God set apart the fruit of this one tree? God had given them a free will and the ability to make choices. Why would we be given a free will if there was not a choice to be made?

God told Adam and Eve to abstain from eating from its fruit because He did not want them to have knowledge of evil. He had given them full knowledge of all He called good.

God calls us in the same way today. Paul wrote to the Philippians, Whatsoever things are true, honest, just, pure, lovely and of good report; if there be any virtue, and if there be any praise, think on these things. (see Philippians 4:8). It is up to us to choose and if we have not renewed our minds, we are still inclined to make the wrong choices.

Look at the children of Israel. Food was an issue with them. It was one of the first things they complained about. "And the children of Israel said to them, 'Oh, that we had died by the hand of the Lord in the land of Egypt, when we sat by the pots of meat and when we ate bread to the full! For you have brought us out into this wilderness to kill this whole assembly with hunger.' Then the Lord said to Moses, 'Behold I will rain bread from heaven for you. And the people shall go out and gather a certain quota every day, that I may test them, whether they will walk in My law or not' " (Exodus 16:3-4). God used food to teach them to be dependent on Him.

What we eat is really not about the number on the scale or the size of clothes we wear, but about the battle in our mind and heart. We need to think about the importance of food in our life—is food more important to us than God? Is food our comfort in time of need? Do we reward ourselves with food? What do we turn to in times of stress, during trials in our life and even in times of happiness? Do we treasure the Word of God? "...I have treasured the words of His mouth more than my necessary food" (Job 23:12). We have a helper, the Holy Spirit to comfort us in our time of need. Are we like the Israelites who were more interested in their physical food than their fellowship with God? "They willfully put God to the test by demanding the food they craved" (NIV Psalm 78:18).

As always Jesus is our example. "As He is, so are we in this world" (1John 4:17). People used to tell me that Jesus was tempted in all ways as I was. I had a hard time seeing Jesus being tempted by a hot fudge sundae! But one day I read, "…He was hungry" (Luke 4:2). I'd read that before, but this time I had a light bulb moment. I understood at a much deeper level that Jesus really did know what it was to be hungry.

Satan used the same tactic on Jesus that he had used on Eve. He appealed to Jesus' physical need for food. Lust of the eyes—the devil promised Jesus entire kingdoms if He would bow to the god of this world. Pride of life— he tried to entice Jesus to prove His significance by forcing God to command angels to save Him.

When Eve was tempted she was in a beautiful garden surrounded by luscious food that she could eat freely. Jesus was in a deprived state from fasting 40 days, yet He overcame the temptation of the enemy! How did He do this? By speaking the truth of God's Word "It is written…" (Luke 4:1-15). With every temptation, Jesus made a choice. He quoted Scripture that exposed the lie of the enemy. Truth is powerful. Jesus said, "And you shall know the truth and the truth shall make you free" (John 8:32). The power comes when we believe what we speak. How did we get saved? We believed with our heart and we spoke with our mouth (Romans 10:10). The words that we spoke out of our mouth had

> The power comes when we believe what we speak.

the power to deliver us from the kingdom of darkness into the kingdom of light.

That is a principle of the Kingdom of Heaven that we continue to use as we walk the runway of life as a child of God. "And since we have the same spirit of faith, according to what is written, 'I believed and therefore I spoke.' We also believe and therefore speak" (2 Corinthians 4:13). We speak what we believe and our faith in God is activated to bring about the deliverance that we need. Deliverance from temptation, deliverance from sickness, depression and oppression of the devil. Deliverance from the fear of rejection and failure. Competition and jealousy, bondage—the list is endless, but the God we serve is bigger than the deception of the enemy.

Notice that Paul said 'a spirit of faith'. Faith comes from our spirit, from inside and as we speak, our faith becomes a reality.

Proverbs has a lot to tell us about the words of our mouth. "You are snared by the words of your mouth; you are taken by the words of your mouth" (Proverbs 6:2). "Death and life are in the power of the tongue, and those who love it will eat its fruit" (Proverbs 18:21). It is awesome to me that by the words of our mouth we are delivered from the kingdom of darkness into the kingdom of light. It is an issue of the heart. Matthews tells us, "…for out of the abundance of the heart the mouth speaks" (Matthew 12:34).

That means what is in our heart is going to come out of our mouth and that can bring death or life. What we put into our heart is our choice. If we feed our heart with the Word of God then our heart will feed our mouth in our time of trouble. Jesus was full of the Word. Jesus walked the earth as a man to teach us and show us the ways of the Kingdom of Heaven. He is our example. When He was tempted by satan, He spoke the Word of God. We must do the same.

It is our job to feed on the Word and renew our mind. As we are renewing our mind, we are also building a strong spirit. "But the Helper, the Holy Spirit, whom the Father will send in My name, He will teach you all things, and bring to your remembrance all things that I said to you" (John 14:26). If the Word is in us the Holy Spirit can bring it to our remembrance in our time of need.

One day I wanted a piece of coconut cream pie. I had visions of the pie dancing through my thoughts. I was remembering just how good it tasted when suddenly I heard, "The Lord is your shepherd you shall not want" (Psalm 23:1). Instantly the craving was gone. This is an example of the ministry of the Holy Spirit. When we place the Word in our heart the Holy Spirit can bring it to our remembrance.

We must recognize who the enemy is and resist the temptation. Satan always tries to make us think that we have to have something to comfort us and then pours on the guilt after we have given in to the temptation. How do we resist? All resistance is based on submission. "Therefore, submit to God. Resist the devil and he will flee from you" (James 4:7). Our ability to resist the devil is proportionate to our submission to the Lord. If we take the time to submit to the Lord in the morning, we will have the ability to resist the devil the rest of the day. We need daily manna from His Word. Just as the Israelites had to gather daily manna for the day, we have to gather fresh manna from His Word every day.

If we are not happy with our lives, then we need to change our choices. We are responsible for the choices we make and the only real assurance we have for tomorrow is the choice we make today.

> If we are not happy with our lives, then we need to change our choices.

As we renew our mind with the Word of God our faith in God becomes strong and we learn to trust Him to work through us. As we change on the inside we will see change on the outside. Happiness is an inside job! We try to change the outside when we don't have reality on the inside! The difference we make with our lives is contingent on the difference we allow God to make in our lives.

"...I have set before you life and death,
blessing and cursing; therefore choose life,
that both you and your descendants may live."

(DEUT. 30:19)

4

Created in His Image

"Then God said, 'Let Us make man in Our image, according to Our likeness; let them have dominion over the fish of the sea, over the birds of the air, and over the cattle, over all the earth and over every creeping thing that creeps on the earth.'"

(GENESIS 1:26)

We have dominion over every creeping thing! Does that mean those creeping pounds that sneak upon us over the years? I hear people casting out calories, but unfortunately, my body counts every calorie even if I don't!

We have been promised a way of escape in 1 Corinthians 10:13, "No temptation has overtaken you except such as is common to man; but God is faithful, who will not allow you to be tempted beyond what you are able; but with the temptation will also make the way of escape; that you may be able to bear it." I believe one

21

route of our escape is to grow in the grace and knowledge of God. Hosea 4:6 tells us, "My people are destroyed for lack of knowledge…" That's you and me. We, the born again children of God must learn His ways.

What does it mean to be created in His image and His likeness? The dictionary tells us that image means—a reproduction of the appearance of someone. Likeness—the state of quality resembling or being like something. Paul says, "Imitate me, just as I also imitate Christ" (1 Corinthians 11:1).

> Understanding gives us a way of escape!

Do we really grasp the meaning of these scriptures? "For In Him we live and move and have our being…"(Acts 17:28). Until we understand who we are and how we function in this world as a born again believer in Jesus Christ, we are going to go around our mountain over and over again. Whether our mountain is weight, alcohol, drugs or sex!

Understanding gives us a way of escape! "God is Spirit, and those who worship Him must worship in spirit and truth." (John 4:24). "Now may the God of peace Himself sanctify you completely; and may your whole spirit, soul, and body be preserved blameless at the coming of our Lord Jesus Christ" (1 Thessalonians 5:23). We are actually a three part being created in His image—spirit, soul and body. As we learn the function of each part we begin to walk in the authority and dominion that God has given us to live in this world. We were not created to merely survive! Our DNA gives us the ability to overcome in this world. "For whatever is born of God overcomes the world. And this is the victory that has overcome the world—our faith" (1 John 5:4). We are born of God and our faith in God will help us overcome anything we face in this world. Our faith comes from our spirit.

Remember we are not waging a battle of the flesh in which we have to exert our will power and self-control. This is spiritual warfare and if we do not learn how to fight in the spirit we are going to be a prisoner of war in satan's camp.

God breathed into Adam and made his soul and body come alive. He put within man a spirit to have communion with Him. Through the spirit we can understand and know the ways of God as we walk in this world just as Adam and Eve could commune with God. Conversion, being born again, gives us the ability to commune with God. As we stated earlier, what Adam and Eve lost in the Garden, Jesus bought back at Calvary. Those that have not accepted Jesus do not know or understand what is going on in a Christian's life. They are on the outside trying to understand. It is only when we can see from the inside through our spiritual eyes that we understand.

The Holy Spirit comes to dwell in our spirit when we are born again. He is our teacher, our counselor, our comforter and He will bring all things to our remembrance. (John 14:25-26). In our spirit we have meaning and purpose in life. Through our spirit we have communion and fellowship with God. Our spirit gives us discernment between right and wrong. Our spiritual health has a significant impact on our emotional health which impacts our physical health. The connection of spirit, soul, and body is extremely important for us to flow in unity with our Father in heaven.

Our soul is what gives us our personality and through our soul we live out our relationships with other people and ourselves. The soul has three major components—our mind, will and emotions. Our mind is where we do our thinking and reasoning. It is also the bed for our emotions, feelings and memories. Our will gives us the ability to make choices. The soul of man is in close relationship with the outside shell, our body. The three areas of the soul help the body to know what to do, when to do it and how to do it.

Our body— that part of us that is seen in the world comes in various shapes, sizes and colors! It is easy for us to classify and identify. The body has five senses — seeing, feeling, smelling, touching and hearing. The body is a wonder to man. Every day scientists discover more truth about the human body. The body holds a remarkable pump, the heart. It works harder and longer than any engine ever made by man. The head contains the human brain which is far beyond medical comprehension. It is our responsibility to care for our body, to nurture it and protect it, as well as the environment in which our body lives. Our body is a sacred garment. We need to treat our body with honor. Our bodies will follow our mind set. The body does not think or make decisions. It is a slave to our soul and our soul needs to be directed by our spirit.

> How can we present our body to God when we have no control over it?

Romans 12:1 tells us, "I beseech you therefore brethren, by the mercies of God, that you present your bodies a living sacrifice, holy, acceptable to God, which is your reasonable service." How can we present our body to God when we have no control over it?

In man we see that he has a spirit, soul and body. Through his soul, he rules the natural things around him. He has emotions to admire the beauty of his surroundings in this earth. He has the willpower to make choices. With his spirit he understands his limitations in this world. He knows what he should do and what he should not do relative to good and evil. His body (or his earth suit) carries the soul and the spirit. "Or do you not know that your body is the temple of the Holy Spirit who is in you, whom you have from God, and you are not your own?" (1 Corinthians

6:19). James tells us, "for as the body without the spirit is dead, so faith without works is dead also" (James 2:26).

Our spirit is king, our soul a servant and our body a slave. Your spirit shows kingship by praising God. There are many times we will not feel like praising God in this world, but our soul and body do not have a choice. Our spirit should rule our thoughts which then should rule our actions. David is a good example for us. We read in the Psalms that he told his soul how to respond. "Why are you cast down, O my soul? And why are you disquieted within me?"(Psalm 42:5). David's spirit was speaking to his soul! The soul and spirit are so tightly woven together that only the Word of God can discern between thought and heart. "For the word of God is living and powerful and sharper than any two-edged sword, piercing even to the division of soul and spirit, and of joints and marrow, and is a discerner of the thoughts and intents of the heart" (Hebrews 4:12).

As a child of God we must become 'spirit' conscious. We must learn to respond from our spirits and not react from our soul —ß our mind, will and emotions. We must bring our spirit into focus to be the king of our life by reading the Word, praying and worshipping.

As we grow in the Word we will become aware of our spirit, soul and body. Psalms 23, a very familiar Psalm states, "...He restores my soul..." Our soul is easily damaged in this world. It is the battle-ground. What we think definitely affects our body and how we make decisions in this world. Romans 12:2 tells us, "And do not be con-formed to this world, but be transformed by the renewing of your mind (soul), that you may prove what is that good and acceptable and perfect will of God." If we want to change habits that have us in bond-age, we must change the way we think first, then our body will follow.

We are told not to be conformed to this world. Conforming to the world's way is allowing the pressure from the outside to shape us and mold us. Transformation comes from inside through the truth of God's Word.

> A strong spirit is not a gift from God; it is something that we build by feeding on the Word, through prayer and fellowship with God.

To change the way we think we must feed on His Word and build a strong spirit. Luke 2:40 tells us, "the Child (Jesus) grew and became strong in spirit, filled with wisdom…" A strong spirit is not a gift from God; it is something that we build by feeding on the Word, through prayer and fellowship with God. The Holy Spirit dwells in our spirit and communicates with our spirit. Our spirit should direct our soul in what we think on and our will in making decisions for our lives. Our emotions should also be controlled by our spirit. Don't forget the joy of the Lord is our strength! (Nehemiah 8:10). If our spirit does not control our soul and our body, the world will. In this 'anything goes' culture of ours the advertising world and the media are just waiting to influence your choices and appetite!

Sad to say, most Christians are living out of their soul. Up one day and down the next. Living by the dictates of the flesh—what feels good at the moment. The world even recognizes 'comfort food' that makes us happy.

"But if the Spirit of Him who raised Jesus from the dead dwells in you, He who raised Christ from the dead will also give life to your mortal bodies through His Spirit who dwells in you" (Romans 8:11). A strong spirit will lead us through life's trials and tribulations giving us peace and an assurance that we are not alone because the Father is with us.

Most of us have an undernourished spirit with our soul stuffed

Most of us have an undernourished spirit with our soul stuffed with the trash of the world.

with the trash of the world. When we focus on the soul and its knowledge from the world and the way the world thinks, we deaden the voice of our spirit. Our spirit is broken. Proverbs 18:14 says, "The spirit of a man will sustain him in sickness, but who can bear a broken spirit?"

Our spirit man must be fed the Word of God. John 6:63 tells us, "It is the Spirit who gives life; the flesh profits nothing. The words that I speak to you are spirit and they are life". God's Word brings light and life.

Proverbs 25:28 gives us insight into the frustrations of life. "Whoever has no rule over his own spirit is like a city broken down without walls." A city without walls lacks clear identity and boundaries. It has no means to protect itself.

If your soul is in control of your life you will not have solid boundaries that can protect you. God designed our spirit to be dominant and the soul to be subordinate to the spirit.

When we are filled with the Spirit and walk in the Spirit as we are told to do in Galatians 5:16, "… walk in the Spirit, and you shall not fulfill the lust of the flesh," the Holy Spirit that is within you infuses your spirit and controls your spirit, soul and body. Your spirit will have the dominance that it was created to have.

When your spirit is in control you will see everything through God's perspective.

When your spirit is in control you will see everything through God's perspective. Centering your thoughts on God's thoughts produce joy and peace taking care of many things such as depression, lies of the enemy that you have believed, discouragement, and comparing yourself with others, including jealousy.

Proverbs is full of verses about our spirit. Chapter 17 verse 22 says, "A merry heart (spirit) does good, like medicine, But a broken spirit dries the bones." Job 32:8 says, "But there is a spirit in man, and the breath of the Almighty gives him understanding." There is a list of scriptures in the back of this book to bring greater revelation about your spirit. Understanding how we function in this world, as a child of God, is of utmost importance in enabling us to walk in the spirit, hear His voice and follow Him.

For too long we have allowed our soul to dominate our spirit. We have believed the lies of the enemy and lived in regret of the past or fantasies about the future. We have allowed the bombardment of the world, the flesh, and the devil to control our thinking.

> For too long we have allowed our soul to dominate our spirit.

As we walk through this world we can't help picking up some dirt. We must continually wash with the water of the Word (Ephesians 5:26) to keep our minds (soul) focused on God and His ways. Isaiah 26:3 tells us, "You will keep him in perfect peace, whose mind is stayed on You, because he trusts in You."

Our Father is always working on our behalf, bringing us to a place of understanding our birthright as a child of God. Christianity is about relationship and fellowship. It is not a religious activity. Our part is to be diligent in the Word of God, to develop a lifestyle of prayer and praise Him for His goodness and faithfulness. I don't understand how it all works, but I do know my responsibility.

People who do not feed their spirit faithfully cannot embrace the fullness of the life that God has prepared for them. They feel isolated, just trudging through this world without purpose, waiting for the sweet by and by. We can be happy living in this world with all its problems because He has given us everything that pertains to life and godliness (2 Peter 1-4).

If we do not learn how to function as a child of God and how to fight the powers of darkness and principalities of the air (Ephesians 6:12) we will fall into the hands of the enemy and it will be easy for the enemy to trap us with addictions to food, drugs, alcohol, sex or pornography.

Many people have received salvation but never understood that salvation includes fullness of life on earth. Saying yes to Jesus opens the door for deliverance and healing in every area of our life— spirit, soul and body.

Your body is unique. You were created and you are not an accident. Your Heavenly Father chose the day and the time your life would begin. Psalms 139:13-16 tells us, "For you created my inmost being; you knit me together in my mother's womb. I praise you because I am fearfully and wonderfully made; your works are wonderful, I know that full well. My frame was not hidden from you when I was made in the secret place, when I was woven together in the depths of the earth. Your eyes saw my unformed body; all the days ordained for me were written in your book before one of them came to be" (NIV).

You are unique, there is nobody like you. God thought a lot about you. Every detail of your body, every cell and organ, are the results of God's thoughts about you. Your personality is His handiwork. God has made an investment in you, giving you gifts and talents to be used for His Glory. He has great joy in His heart as He watches over you.

> Every detail of your body, every cell and organ, are the results of God's thoughts about you.

29

The world needs you. You bring something to the world that no one else has. We must take care of our body and not abuse it by over eating, or becoming addicted to anything but His Word.

> When the purpose for our body becomes a revelation to us, we will no longer abuse it.

There is a purpose for the body. When the purpose for our body becomes a revelation to us, we will no longer abuse it. Our body is the temple of the Holy Spirit (1 Cor. 6:19). The body is the vehicle that God uses to carry the good news into the world. Our body carries the spirit which is fed through our soul and gives voice to the Holy Spirit.

The enemy does not want you taking care of your body. The devil wants you fat! He knows that you will then be open for disease that will steal, kill and destroy Gods purpose for you.

We can be happy in this earth, even walking through the trials of life. Life is full of pain, but misery is optional for the child of God. Paul tells us in Ephesians that we are to be, "praying always with all prayer and supplication in the Spirit, being watchful to this end with all perseverance and supplication for all the saints" (Ephesians 6:18). Praying in the spirit is one of our weapons of warfare. You are building yourself up in your most holy faith praying in the Holy Spirit according to Jude.

Jude 20 tells us the best way to maintain your life with God, "But you, beloved, building yourselves up on your most holy faith praying in the Holy Spirit." In Romans we read, "Likewise the Spirit also helps in our weaknesses. For we do not know what we should pray for as we ought, but the Spirit Himself makes intercession for us with groining's which cannot be uttered" (Romans 8:26). Paul tells us that, "For if I pray in a tongue, my spirit prays, but my understanding is unfruitful" (1 Corinthians 14:14). When we feel confused, frightened or upset about something in our life, we can release our spirit, by praying in the spirit. Praying in the spirit gives voice to our spirit. The peace and calm that results makes it possible for us to hear God's voice and direction.

As we mentioned before—this is not just another diet plan but a battle plan. It is spiritual warfare because the enemy is fighting for our lives. Whatever bondage he can get us in, he is after one thing, our very life. Remember he comes to steal, kill and destroy! (John 10:10). He wants us miserable and he wants to destroy our testimonies as children of God.

1 Corinthians 12:1 states, "Now concerning spiritual gifts brethren, I do not want you to be ignorant." The nine gifts of the Spirit are given to us so the Holy Spirit can help us in our time of need. We need a word of wisdom, a word of knowledge and discerning of spirits in our everyday lives. Because we are fighting a spiritual battle we need to discern the spirit that is coming against us. A word of wisdom or knowledge will enable us to cut asunder the thick cords of the enemy. It is well worth our time to study these specific gifts of the Spirit. We shouldn't turn down a 'gift' from God just because we don't understand it. When we ask the Holy Spirit to teach us He will lead us to a Scripture, a book, a person, or a church to learn what we need to know. Chapter 12 of 1 Corinthians ends by saying, "But earnestly desire the best gifts. And yet I show you a more excellent way." The Holy Spirit will not push us; they are gifts to receive, but we must earnestly desire these gifts.

"The light of the eyes rejoices the heart, and a good report makes the bones healthy" (Proverbs 15:30). When light (understanding) comes to your soul, your spirit rejoices and your body responds!

> As our mind is renewed our spirit is fed, we receive revelation and our body will do what it is told to do!

When your spirit, soul and body are in unity, there is nothing that can stop you from your plans and purposes.

This is a life time learning experience. As our mind is renewed our spirit is fed, we receive revelation and our body will do what it is told to do!

What has this to do with weight loss? You need the power of the Holy Spirit within your spirit to break the strongholds in your mind (soul) that trigger your taste buds. You need help from the power within you to fight the rejections and fears that trigger the deception of your need for comfort food.

I urge you to study the spirit, soul and body continually so you grow in your understanding of how you were created to function in this world as a child of God. We must feed our soul to strengthen our spirit and renew our mind. A healthy well fed Christian can resist the attacks of the enemy much easier.

Knowledge is a way of escape from the pain of this life on earth. One resource I highly recommend is a book by Lester Sumrall—Spirit, Soul and Body. It explains in depth how the spirit, soul and body work individually and together.

"The entrance of Your words gives light; It gives understanding to the simple."

(PSALM 119:130)

5

The Battle of the Bulge

"For the weapons of our warfare are not carnal but mighty in God for pulling down strongholds, casting down arguments and every high thing that exalts itself against the knowledge of God, bringing every thought into captivity to the obedience of Christ."

(2 CORINTHIANS 10:4-5)

In every battle you face you must know who your enemy is, how he thinks and how he operates. Our enemy is satan and he has only one weapon—deception.

I have quoted this scripture before, but it bears repeating. "But I fear, lest somehow, as the serpent deceived Eve by his craftiness, so your mind may be corrupted from the simplicity that is in Christ" (2 Corinthian 11:3).

Eve fell prey when she considered satan's suggestion. She knew the tree was forbidden, but when she looked at the tree again *after* thinking about satan's idea, it seemed different. It would benefit her and it looked delicious! What would one little bite hurt? Satan can only work by suggestions; he cannot force us to do anything. If we give in to his thought, it is only because we chose to do so. This is his plan, that we make a choice of our own free will then we feel guilty after giving in to our appetite. He has hit us with a double whammy! Making a bad decision followed with guilt.

Satan is clever, his suggestions are so subtle that he can take thoughts that we know are wrong and make them appear to be right. For example he can deceive us into thinking the more we eat the more satisfied we will be. We eat unhealthy food, become fat and dis-satisfied, but return to the refrigerator for more.

We have thousands of thoughts in a day, but we do not have to think on every thought we have. Our mind is the battlefield. We are told to cast down every thought and imagination that is against the knowledge of God's Word. To do this we must know the Word of God.

> We have thousands of thoughts in a day, but we do not have to think on every thought we have.

The Bible tells us, "Let this mind be in you which was also in Christ Jesus" (Philippians 2:5). How do we know God? Through the knowledge of the Word of God which renews our mind. We accept God's ideas in our mind and we call this inspiration. Satan works to get us to accept his ideas and suggestions and that is called temptation. Whatever idea we accept, whether from God or satan, it controls our behavior. This should be no surprise to us. The devil is a master counterfeiter.

Jesus told His disciples in Mark 8:15 to be aware of the leaven of the Pharisees. Leaven is a subtle influence that alters the way you think. Satan floats ideas into our mind when we least expect it. When we continue to think on these thoughts they become strongholds. A stronghold is a group of thoughts that control our reasoning. These strongholds are built over time and we are not aware of what is going on.

Satan begins to form patterns of thoughts early in our life with nagging thoughts, fears, suspicions, and reasoning. Habits are formed from strongholds in our mind. When something becomes a habit it takes very little conscious effort to take action. How often do we "automatically" pop a piece of candy into our mouth or eat an extra piece of cake without giving any thought to it? That is a stronghold working in our mind and feeding our habit to eat without even thinking about it. Our emotions and feelings are triggered inside us by the habit patterns we've established over time.

> Habits are formed from strongholds in our mind.

I remember flying home from a meeting once. When I stepped out of the airplane, immediately I was transfixed by the delicious aroma of caramel corn. I didn't even give it a thought, I just followed the smell! After stuffing my face, I felt guilty and ashamed. I gave no thought to the calories that I just ate! Whoever said calories don't count listened to a lie of the devil! You might not count calories, but your body counts every calorie that goes into your mouth and it ends up some place on your body in ugly fat. It all started by one little suggestion that I couldn't resist.

We must start thinking about what we are thinking about! If we are going to stop this merry-go-round, we must become aware of our enemy, guard our thoughts, ask ourselves where the thought came from and simply refuse to accept the ideas that satan tries to plant in our mind.

We must be alert for the temptation and become aware of the trigger points in our lives. Discouraging thoughts come against me and immediately my stomach kicks in sending a message to my brain that I need comfort food. We receive bad news. We compare ourselves with someone else. We have a fear of rejection and failure. We are jealous and allow bitterness to come into our life. These are just a few of the devil's devices to keep us self-centered and thinking about ourselves.

You just sit down to relax and watch TV and a commercial break comes on. Without thinking you get up and go to the kitchen. You look in the fridge, nothing there, go to the cabinet, then back to the fridge like something just materialized there in the last 30 seconds! You have to learn to recognize your first food thought! You are not hungry, it is a habit!

Paul warns us in Ephesians 4:22-23, "Strip yourselves of your former nature—put off and discard your old unrenewed self—which characterized your previous manner of life and becomes corrupt through lusts and desires that spring from delusion; and be constantly renewed in the spirit of your mind—having a fresh mental and spiritual attitude." (Amplified) This is the way of life for the child of God. As we walk the runway of life there are always temptations to overcome, but as our souls prosper, we will have an automatic response from our mouth that will drive satan crazy!

The Bible says that all resistance is based on submission. "Therefore submit to God, resist the devil and he will flee from you" (James 4:7). He has no choice. You have the choice. How did Jesus resist the devil when He was tempted with hunger? (Luke 4:2). He spoke to the devil. Every time the devil tempted Jesus, He spoke the word of God. Jesus is our example and you must do the same. You have been given the authority (Luke 10:19). The enemy does not give up easily, but as you submit yourself to God and His word you will become aware of the way he operates and be able to resist his temptations.

When his thought strikes, speak to it! Yes, speak out loud. "No devil, I'm not hungry! I will not bow my knee to your temptation." Stop the thought before it gains power in your mind and you start to meditate on it.

God desires that we prosper in every area of our lives. He came to give us life. We can be happy living in this world! 3 John 1:2 says, "Beloved, I pray that you may prosper in all things and be in health just as your soul prospers." We studied before that your soul is your mind, will and emotions. I think of it as the soul being the connector between the spirit and body. As you renew your mind with the Word of God, you are also feeding your spirit. This is how you build a strong spirit that can withstand the fiery darts of the enemy! Your body will respond speaking words of faith.

> Stop the thought before it gains power in your mind and you start to meditate on it.

A word is an expression and a fulfillment of a thought. Proverbs tells us that, "You are snared by the words of your mouth; you are taken by the words of your mouth" (Proverbs 6:2) and Proverbs 18:21 says, "Death and life are in the power of the tongue, and those who love it will eat its fruit." Words are powerful; they bring life or death to a situation you are facing in your life. Matthew 12:34 says, "…for out of the abundance of the heart the mouth speaks." What is in our heart will come out our mouth. So if I want to guard what comes out my mouth, I need to be especially careful about what goes into my heart through my soul.

> A word is an expression and a fulfillment of a thought.

As a child of God our soul (mind) longs for God. "As the deer pants for the water brooks, so pants my soul (mind) for You,

O God. My soul thirsts for God, for the living God..." (Psalm 42:1-2a). If we fail to satisfy our soul, then our body will take over, trying to bring comfort with temporary physical pleasures. We must learn the significance of 'fresh manna' every day. There was a reason the Lord only allowed the children of Israel to gather fresh manna daily. Every day brings new challenges; yesterday's manna was for yesterday's challenges. Remember His mercies are new every day (Lamentations 3:23). This is a daily walk. As we walk we must be constantly aware we have an enemy whose focus is to steal, kill and destroy! We must be alert at all times. Isaiah 26:3 says, "You will keep him in perfect peace, whose mind is stayed on You, because he trusts in You."

> We can clearly see that the mind is the forerunner of our actions.

We can clearly see that the mind is the forerunner of our actions. "For those who are according to the flesh and controlled by its unholy desires, set their minds on and pursue those things which gratify the flesh, but those who are according to the Spirit and are controlled by the desires of the Spirit, set their minds on and seek those things which gratify the (Holy) Spirit" (Romans 8:5 Amplified). Our actions are a direct result of what we think.

Jesus told his disciples, "I have food to eat of which you do not know" (John 4:32). What are you craving? You are what you eat in the natural and in the spirit. In the natural you get hungry when you don't eat. In the spirit you get hungry by eating. The more God's Word becomes light to you, the more you want to consume it. Proverbs, the book of wisdom says, "The righteous eats to the satisfying of his soul (mind), but the stomach of the wicked shall be in want" (13:25).

We all know scriptures that bring conviction to us and we usually stay away from them. We don't meditate on them day and night as instructed in Joshua 1:8. That is why we are in bondage to food. When we meditate on the scriptures we make our way prosperous. God has provided what it takes for prosperity in all areas of our life—spirit, soul and body, but we have to follow the instructions.

I read a scripture in Philippians one day that I immediately skipped over, but the Holy Spirit would not let me forget it. It said, "Whose end is destruction, whose god is their belly, and whose glory is in their shame—who set their mind on earthly things" (3:19). Wow, that hits hard! I really did not want to think about this. We must be honest with ourselves. We must allow the Holy Spirit to convict us so that we can turn away from the sin and change our ways.

We become so obsessed in our thought life with food that we refuse to deny our flesh. Our mind is determined to have what feels good for the moment. Our mind is always saying—I want, I think, I feel! The soul of man is always seeking its own self-interest and cravings for carnal gratification. If you do not master your soul it will control you.

> We become so obsessed in our thought life with food that we refuse to deny our flesh.

Remember what John said, "Beloved, I pray that you may prosper in all things and be in health, just as your soul prospers" (1 John 3:2). As your soul—your mind, will, and emotions prospers, you will be transformed and prosper in all areas of your life, spirit, soul and body.

The world tells us to be comforted by food, but the Word of God tells us that the Holy Spirit is our comforter. Food can fill our stomachs but never satisfy our souls. The definition of comfort food is: food consumed to improve emotional status, whether to relieve negative psychological affect or to increase positive feeling. Ponder this a moment. It says food is to take away the blues, make us feel better and give us comfort. Only the Holy Spirit can bring comfort and give us joy and peace to face the challenges in life. The enemy has deceived us into thinking that running to food will solve our problems. And yet, we find the real result is out of control eating, obesity and poor health; sometimes leading to an early death.

Food can fill our stomachs but never satisfy our souls.

Remember, food is not our enemy, satan is.

We must break the power of the enemy in our mind regarding food. Breaking the consuming and deceiving thoughts about food in our mind will allow us to make good decisions regarding food for our body, food that will nourish us and give us the strength and energy to face each challenge of our life. Remember, it was food that brought the downfall of man. Food is necessary for our nutrition; we must have it. Thus, it is the perfect tool for satan to use to mislead us. Food is innocent in and of itself. Remember, food is not our enemy, satan is. As our soul prospers and strongholds are torn down, we will overcome this battle in our life. Remember, this battle is not about the number on the scale or the dress size; it is about our relationship with God. God is asking us, just as He asked Adam and Eve in the garden, "Where are you?"

The battle has been won; we must learn to walk in the victory that has been provided. If we want to change our lifestyle, we must first change the way we think. As our soul (mind) prospers, our body will follow.

"...for this purpose the Son of God was manifested, that He might destroy the works of the devil."

(1 JOHN 3:8B)

6

You've Been Around this Mountain Long Enough!

"And the Lord spoke to me, saying:
'You have skirted this mountain long enough;
turn northward'."

(DEUTERONOMY 2:2-3)

It is much easier to live in a rut than to break a habit! But we each must come to the place where enough is enough and declare satan has tormented me and stolen from me long enough!

I believe you are ready or you would not be reading this book. I have been around this mountain for years. I would start the journey and then get side tracked. I was busy working for the Lord; I didn't have time to take care of myself.

Is that not deception in the first degree? Satan is not stupid and he watches us, our actions, and learns our weak moments. It is in our physical weakness that he is able to plant just one thought at a time.

> As a child of God you are not designed to walk alone.

One thing I have learned in my life is that crisis is normal to life. We must be prepared to face crisis and not allow it to turn our direction back southward. It is time to go north and we cannot do this on our own. As a child of God you are not designed to walk alone. You are created in His image, you are made for fellowship. God loved to walk in the garden with Adam and Eve and fellowship with them. This is where the enemy struck. He cut off the fellowship and communication. When God asked the question, "Where are you," he was not asking about their place in the garden, but about their relationship with Him.

I love reading the book of John as Jesus was preparing to leave his disciples. He was pouring out His heart to them, knowing what they were going to face. The hardest part of my life as a missionary was standing at the airport with my children getting ready to fly across the world. I would pour out my heart giving all that motherly advice I felt they needed at my departure. Unfortunately we didn't have email and Skype then and international telephone calls were very expensive so communication was not easy. I can still see that look on their faces. Yes, mother, we've heard this all before! As a child of God we can have this same attitude. I read that once, I know what I'm supposed to do. I've heard that sermon before, too bad so and so is not here to hear it. Guess what, we are the ones those messages are intended for.

As Jesus is pouring out his heart to the disciples one of the most significant things that He reminds them of is that they are not alone.

They don't have to face the world on their own. "Nevertheless I tell you the truth, It is to your advantage that I go away, for if I do not go away, the Helper will not come to you; but if I depart, I will send Him to you" (John 16:7). We have an advantage over this world! We have a helper, the Holy Spirit, to help in our time of need.

"These things I have spoken to you while being present with you. But the Helper, the Holy Spirit whom the Father will send in My name, He will teach you all things, and bring to your remembrances all things that I said to you. Peace I leave with you. My peace I give to you; not as the world gives do I give to you. Let not your heart be troubled, neither let it be afraid" (John 14:25-27).

The Holy Spirit is our teacher and He will bring to our remembrance in our time of need the Word that will bring deliverance to us for that specific situation. If we have not read and put the Word of God in our soul, the Holy Spirit cannot bring it to our remembrance. Our remembrance is part of our mind (soul). This is where we think and make decisions. We must decide whose report we will believe. Will we receive the Word brought to us by the Holy Spirit, or will we allow the thief to kill, steal and destroy? "It is the Spirit who gives life; the flesh profits nothing. The words that I speak to you are spirit, and they are life" (John 6:63). God's word brings strength to us. Our faith is strengthened by the Word of God and gives us the confidence to ask for help.

So many times when I have been facing a crisis I have heard that still small voice that brought deliverance. At a time of crisis, the tendency is for fear and panic to immediately take over. That is the moment; the spirit in you must rise and receive from the Holy Spirit. I went to the doctor a while back for a routine physical examination and the doctor said, "I have a bad report for you." For just a moment, I felt fear, then I heard, "He sent His Word to heal you." I didn't know where that word was in the Bible, I did not remember reading it. But sometime I had read it and the Holy Spirit was bringing it to my remembrance. I immediately grabbed that Word and kept saying it out loud! "He sent His word to heal me!" Yes, out loud in the doctor's office in front of the nurse and doctor. Yes, they looked at me as if I was nuts.

> At a time of crisis, the tendency is for fear and panic to immediately take over.

This was my life, I didn't need a bad report and I had a Word from God. I was not letting go of it. My head was already trying to fill my mind with worry and doubt. I was in the middle of a battle. The doctor said, "You have a lump in your breast and under your arm." My head was saying, "too bad this has happened to you. You are a good wife and mother." I was in a battle for my life and I refused to give up my Word. I said it out loud, because my head needed to hear my mouth speaking the Words.

The doctor said, "I suppose you are one of those born again believers who believes in miracles?" "Yes!" I shouted. I left the doctor's office refusing to speak to anyone. I had to get this Word settled in my heart. I could not allow the enemy to steal the Word. When I arrived at my own office and opened the door I saw the Daily Bread devotional book on my desk. I opened it for the day and read, "...I am the Lord who heals all your disease..." (Psalm 103:3). Needless to say, I had a glory fit right then and there! I knew I was healed. When I returned for my appointment for x-rays and biopsy, the lump was gone! This is the God I serve! You put the Word of God in you and the Holy Spirit will bring it to your remembrance in your time of need.

Romans 15:4 tells us, "For whatever things were written before were written for our learning, that we through the patience and comfort of the Scriptures might have hope." The Bible is not just a book of stories. It is a book of testimonies describing how God delivered His people from the snare of the enemy. We can learn from their examples—good and bad.

God brought the children of Israel out to bring them in! He brought them out of bondage to bring them into a land flowing with milk and honey. When the Lord brought them out of Egypt, He told them that He would not give them the land flowing with milk and honey in one year, but that He would drive out the enemy little by little as they increased (Exodus 23: 29–30). They came out of Egypt with a slave mentality. They were not ready to overtake the enemy. They had to learn to recognize their enemy, know how to defeat him, and maintain the victory!

We are not going to win this battle over night. We have all wanted to lose 50 pounds while we are sleeping. Our deliverance will come as we increase in revelation and understanding. The promise of God will be firmly established in our heart and there is no demon in hell that will be able to rob us of our victory!

We have believed the lie of the enemy long enough. It is time to ask, seek and knock that the Lord would reveal His strategy to us so that we will have the wisdom and understanding to overcome this temptation in our lives.

"Let no one say when he is tempted 'I am tempted by God, for God cannot be tempted by evil, nor does He Himself tempt anyone'" (James 1:13). James starts by telling us, "My brethren, count it all joy when you fall into various trials, knowing that the testing of your faith produces patience" (James 1:2-3). We see that as we are in the world there will be various trials.

Trials can be in relationships, finances, health—all those things that effect our lives in the world. Testing is in the spirit. It is a testing of our faith and faith is a spiritual force. There is a difference between a test and a trial. A test is in the spirit, a trial is in the natural world. God does test the heart of man. "The refining pot is for silver and the furnace for gold, but the Lord tests the hearts" (Proverbs 17:3). The purpose of a test is to make us dependent on God.

> The purpose of a test is to make us dependent on God.

"Blessed is the man who endures temptation; for when he has been approved, he will receive the crown of life which the Lord has promised to those who love Him." (James 1:12). It is not the man that endures the trial, but the man who endures the temptation! The temptation to the child of God is to doubt God's Word.

> The temptation to the child of God is to doubt God's Word.

"But each one is tempted when he is drawn away by his own desires and enticed, then, when desire has conceived, it gives birth to sin; and sin, when it is full-grown, brings forth death. Do not be deceived, my beloved brethren" (vs. 14-16). When we give in to the temptation to eat when we are not hungry or to eat food that is not healthy for us, then the enemy brings forth guilt and condemnation. If we continue this year after year then our health is destroyed and even death can be the end result.

When I started this journey with the word from God, "break the habit," I had no idea how hard it was going to be.

I was praying and seeking the Lord asking for help, I heard another word. "Fasting is the gateway to the supernatural". Fasting had never been a habit of mine. I was brought up in a very religious home where you fasted to get God to move. If He didn't then you got mad at Him.

I had not heard a lot of teaching on fasting, maybe just a mention every now and then.

After receiving this Word from the Lord, I knew I had to search the scriptures about fasting. When we receive a word from the Lord, it is our responsibility to continue seeking for revelation. We will not walk in the fulfillment of the Word until we have understanding and revelation of the purpose of the Word. There is always a purpose for a Word from the Lord!

I learned that fasting was to move us, so that God could move. The stronghold in my mind was not going to come down easily. Satan had gained dominion over my body through my appetite. He had gained access to my will. When we try to dislodge the enemy from his base of operation we have a war on our hands. We need every spiritual weapon that is available and if Jesus fasted to defeat the enemy, then I think we can safely say that we need to fast as we prepare for battle.

It is time to break the habit, get out of the rut and take a new direction that will not lead us around the same old mountain of defeat!

"Show me Your ways, O Lord, teach me Your paths. Lead me in Your truth and teach me. For you are the God of my salvation, On You I wait all the day."

(Psalm 25:4-5)

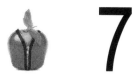 **7**

Fasting: the Weapon of Choice

***"Is this not the fast that I have chosen:
to loose the bonds of wickedness, to undo the
heavy burdens, to let the oppressed go free.
And that you break every yoke?"***

(ISAIAH 58:6)

This verse summed it up! I was under a yoke of bondage. The bonds of wickedness had placed a heavy burden and brought me under the oppression of the enemy. I needed help; I could not break this on my own.

God chose fasting and prayer as a way for us to set ourselves apart from the distractions of this world. Read Isaiah 58 and ask the Lord to speak to you and open the eyes of your understanding to break the habits that hold you in bondage and lift the oppression that keeps you from enjoying your freedom in Christ.

Fasting is renouncing the natural to invoke the supernatural. The most natural thing to do is eat. In fasting we don't change God's mind, but we begin to understand God's heart. When we fast we are deliberately turning away from the natural and looking to the supernatural. We are humbling ourselves before God and admitting our need.

> When we fast we are deliberately turning away from the natural and looking to the supernatural.

In Isaiah 58 there are four main reasons to fast and pray: losing the bonds of wickedness, undoing the heavy burden, letting the oppressed go free and breaking every yoke.

The bonds of wickedness refer to such things as sinful habits—including self-inflicted bad habits, addictions, and spiritual strongholds. We need to face the rebellion in our life that caused the addiction, habit, obsession or compulsion.

A person bound in wickedness has a false perception of reality. He is so bound that he cannot respond to the love of God and His forgiveness and mercy. His thought life is centered on his addiction, seeking revenge or feeding his habit. Only the Holy Spirit can bring deliverance to this person.

Living in this world today is not easy. The world is becoming darker every day and we must now more than ever learn to trust the Lord with our daily lives. It is easy to get weighed down by life's problems. Job says, "Man that is born of a woman is of few days, and full of trouble" (Job 14:1). Many people are suffering today from financial burdens. Sometimes a person carrying a heavy burden feels hopeless and takes on too many responsibilities causing him to feel a burden. We allow others to place circumstances on us that cause us to feel bogged down and unhappy. Disease in our body can cause a burden. God desires that we be delivered from these burdens of life.

As we fast and pray we must seek God for a word of wisdom and clear direction for the way of escape. Seek the wise counsel of others. No one can bear their burden alone.

People feel oppressed when they feel trapped in a situation and see no purpose in their life. Oppression is a spiritual condition rooted in unbelief. Always depressed with no joy in their life, they are miserable and make everyone around them miserable! Oppression usually results from how we perceive something, rather than the actual circumstances. At the heart of oppression is fear and anxiety which stem from our inability to believe that God loves us and that God has provided everything we need for this life. "As His divine power has given to us all things that pertain to life and godliness through the knowledge of Him who called us by glory and virtue" (2 Peter 1:3).

God has promised all things that pertain to life and godliness! The oppressed person always wants to flee, to run from the problem. Notice the scripture says, 'through the knowledge'. That means we have to read the Word of God and then we can receive understanding. As we read the Word of God, hope rises in our hearts, feeding our faith and we will see the deliverance of our oppression.

When a person has a yoke of bondage he is constrained by a person or situation. A farmer places a yoke on oxen so they can't escape and must do what he wants. Today a yoke of bondage is generally caused by being in relationships, associations or environments that constrain and cause you to

> As we fast, God may reveal a deeper problem that needs to be healed.

do something that is outside God's will for you. It could be going along with the crowd or allowing peer pressure to control you. People in relationships with abusers are under a yoke of bondage. Galatians 5:1 tells us, "Stand fast therefore in the liberty by which

Christ has made us free, and do not be entangled again with a yoke of bondage." We have been set free from the ways of the world which held us in bondage. Paul is warning us not to go back into the ways of the world. There is a better way for the child of God.

Isaiah 58 is aimed at bringing us into a spiritual wholeness. As you read this chapter over and over ask the Holy Spirit to open the eyes of your understanding to the importance of this spiritual weapon.

In this book we are dealing with the food issue, whether it is eating too much or making poor choices, or both. As we fast, God may reveal a deeper problem that needs to be healed. There may be an issue dealing with old rejection and hurts from childhood. Some of us may be under stress from family situations, work or a feeling of unworthiness. The Holy Spirit will reveal the truth to us by stripping away layers of pain and helping us see the excuses we have made to justify our situation.

> A fast is always to draw us into a deeper relationship with God.

A fast is always to draw us into a deeper relationship with God. Seeking God's will for our life is the priority in a time of prayer and fasting. Fasting demands that we confront specific things in our lives—our habits and our relationship with the Lord.

When I began to fast, I asked the Holy Spirit to search my heart. The Holy Spirit began to reveal to me areas of anger and resentment that I had allowed to build a wall around my heart. I had buried the pain of rejection and became rebellious in my attitude.

People had judged me by my appearance and I developed an "I'll show them" attitude. I didn't need them. I had been tripped up by the imperfections in people. I learned that I had to guard my robe of righteousness. I could not allow my robe to come unraveled by my attitude. As we walk the runway of life it is very hard not to pick up some dirt along the way. We must continually guard our heart with all diligence by washing with the water of the word. Our sins are forgiven by the blood of Jesus, but we must constantly wash away the dirt of the world by the water of the Word. (Ephesians 5:26).

As I saw what was in my heart and repented there was a new found freedom and joy in my life. A fasted lifestyle, fasting regularly, helps keep your attitude and heart right.

As we study God's Word we can find many examples of fasting in the Old and New Testament; it is usually always mentioned in conjunction with prayer. Fasting deals with the physical nature of man. Prayer is a spiritual discipline. Prayer turns our eyes toward God and away from the world. What is revealed to us in our time of fasting should become our prayer focus. When we know the focus of our prayer we enter into spiritual warfare. When we obtain breakthrough in prayer and fasting it changes us from the inside out! Victory belongs to us, the enemy is defeated by the power of the Holy Spirit and we are free to enjoy the blessings of our salvation provided by Christ Jesus.

> When we obtain breakthrough in prayer and fasting, it changes us from the inside out!

We must remember that Jesus walked in this world as a man. He ministered by the power of the Holy Spirit. Two things happened in His life before He entered His public ministry. First, the Holy Spirit descended upon Him and He was endued with the supernatural power of the Holy Spirit. Then before going out for His public ministry, He was led by the Spirit into the wilderness and tempted for forty days by the devil. (Luke 4:1-14) In those days he ate nothing and focused on the spiritual. He had face to face experiences of temptation by satan. His fasting prepared Him for battle and for victory over His enemy. We need to notice an important fact of this testimony. When Jesus was led into the wilderness "he was filled with the Holy Spirit" (verse1); the result of fasting was, "Jesus returned to Galilee in the power of the Spirit…" (verse 14). From the time Jesus was baptized, the Spirit was there. But it was His fasting that released the power of the Holy Spirit to overcome the temptation of the enemy. Significant also is the fact in verse 13, "Now when the devil had ended every temptation, he departed from Him until an opportune time." Satan didn't plan to give up, he would watch for a time of weakness to attack again. Remember, "…Your adversary the devil walks about like a roaring lion, seeking whom he may devour" (1 Peter 5:8). Living a fasted lifestyle keeps you sensitive and alert to the deception of the enemy and helps you avoid the pitfalls of life.

Jesus not only fasted, He taught His disciples to fast. Matthew 6:16-18, "Moreover, when you fast, do not be like the hypocrites, with a sad countenance. For they disfigure their faces that they may appear to men to be fasting. Assuredly, I say to you they have their reward. But you, when you fast, anoint your head and wash your face, so that you do not appear to men to be fasting, but to your Father who is in the secret place; and your Father who sees in secret will reward you openly." Here we see Jesus said, "When you fast." He expected them to fast.

Jesus did not give any specific instructions of how long or how often to fast. Fasting was to be a private matter between the person and the Lord. He taught his disciples not to appear to the world to be fasting. The above scripture tells us the hypocrites did that and what people thought of them would be their

> Fasting is a matter of the heart and must be directed by the Holy Spirit.

reward. We also see that God associates fasting with reward and that our reward will be made openly.

Another example is in Matthew 17 where the disciples come to Jesus asking why they could not cast out a demon. "Because of your unbelief......However, this kind does not go out except by prayer and fasting" (vs. 14-21). Jesus clearly indicates that the demonic spirit in this young man could not be cast out because of their unbelief. He then states that this kind can only be cast out through prayer and fasting. I personally believe that we can be so bound by the bonds of wickedness that we must be willing to sacrifice in the natural to find the spiritual power to break the stronghold of the enemy.

Fasting is a matter of the heart and must be directed by the Holy Spirit. As I mentioned, the Lord spoke to my heart, "fasting is the gateway to the supernatural" and I knew that I had to seek the Lord and learn from His Word about fasting.

We all eat much more than our bodies actually need. When we change our food habits, our cravings stop. We crave what we eat. Can any of us eat just one potato chip? I have a very busy schedule and I was constantly picking up fast food loaded with sugar and fat. Fasting broke this habit.

> Fasting brought me to a place of knowing what real hunger was compared to what I perceived hunger to be.

My taste buds were no longer in charge and my body was not in control of my eating habits. I was actually thinking about what I was eating! That's right, before I was mindlessly eating whatever was handy and would stop the craving I was feeling at the moment. Now I am conscious of what I eat and actually take time to plan and prepare.

Preparation is a way of escape from the merry-go-round of over eating. Fasting brought me to a place of knowing what real hunger was compared to what I perceived hunger to be. I was eating out of a habit. My head would say it is time to eat. The real problem I was facing was in my mind. When I was fasting for 10 days, I found it amazing that I continued to think about food, but I was not hungry and had no desire to eat. It became very clear I had been eating from habit and emotions. When I began to feel hunger I knew that it was real and that I was to break the fast.

Since beginning this walk with the Lord I have fasted several times for 10 days drinking only water. I have found when the fast is directed by the Holy Spirit I have not been hungry, but when I tried to do it on my own I was always hungry and couldn't do it. Another thing that has been very helpful to me was a Daniel Fast. This is a fast that has been a great help in learning to control my appetite. (I have listed a book in the recommended reading section about the Daniel fast that was very helpful.) I don't have a set pattern, but I have found that living a fasted lifestyle has many benefits. I find that I am more sensitive to the Holy Spirit and hearing the voice of the Lord. Discernment of what is going on around me is much clearer since I began this lifestyle.

Everyone has weak areas in their lives and I believe that a consistent life of prayer and fasting will alert us to those areas. I have done some pretty dumb things in my life, some of which I have shared with you in this book. God has given me the grace and mercy to overcome my bad eating habits and is renewing my strength day by day. I believe I am stronger and much more effective for the gospel at this time of my life than ever before. I am looking forward to years of serving Him in the ministry and enjoying my great grandchildren in the future. We have eternal life, so what are a few years on this earth?

As I've said before, food has been an issue since the beginning of time. Food addictions, anorexia, bulimia, and obesity are all eating conditions that the devil uses to steal, kill and destroy. And there is the fact that we are constantly buying new clothes to fit the current size and paying for diets and diet pills—all of which rob our finances.

When we master the food issue in our lives we gain much more than losing weight. The joy and happiness that comes from obedience fills our soul. We have emotional stability and know, with the help of the Holy Spirit, that we can walk in obedience.

> When we master the food issue in our lives we gain much more than losing weight.

Why should we fast? The Bible teaches it and Jesus did it. Is there a better reason? The Word of God has much to say about fasting and prayer including the Lord's commands to fast ("when you fast"). You can find many testimonies in the Bible of people fasting and praying using different types of fasts for different reasons. What the Bible teaches us directly and by example is surely something we should do if we want spiritual breakthroughs in our lives.

Fasting brings a fresh anointing, renewed spiritual strength and freshness to our souls.

Fasting is a choice. Fasting is the gateway to the supernatural—breaking out of the routine of life to draw nearer to God.

"So shall I keep Your law continually. Forever and ever. And I will walk at liberty, for I seek Your precepts."

(PSALM 119:44-45)

8

Nothing Tastes As Good As Obedience

"...obedience is better than sacrifice..."

(1 Samuel 15:22b)

Trust and obey, for there's no other way to be happy in Jesus, but to trust and obey. The words of this hymn say it all. As a child of God we must trust that God is for us and that He is working out all things that concern us for our good. When we have confidence in Him, then we will obey and receive the promise which has great reward. Hebrews 10:35 tells us, "Therefore do not cast away your confidence, which has great reward."

As you walk in obedience the joy and peace that comes is better than the weight loss! The weight loss is just an added benefit. Obedience brings contentment to our lives. "Beloved, if our heart does not condemn us, we have confidence toward God" (1 John 3:21).

Joyce Tilney

As a child of God you know immediately in your heart when you have done something wrong. "...Happy is he who does not condemn himself in what he approves" (Romans 14:22b). When we know what God desires of us and are disobedient, the devil does not have to put a guilt trip on us because we condemn ourselves. We have a choice to walk in obedience or to disobey. We must remember that something that is not right for us may be okay for someone else. "Therefore, to him who knows to do good and does not do it, to him it is sin" (James 4:17). This is a personal walk and you have to be obedient to what God is saying to you for your life.

> We must remember that something that is not right for us may be okay for someone else.

We all have areas that we are struggling in. One scripture that I have found helpful to meditate on is, "Everything is permissible for me—but not everything is beneficial. Everything is permissible for me—but I will not be mastered by anything" (1 Corinthians 6:12 NIV). Food is not sin in itself, but when food controls us it can lead us away from God because it becomes more important to us than God. This is called idolatry, which is sin. We seek first food instead of the kingdom of God! We must have food for nutrition, its intended purpose. When we use food for comfort and an emotional pick-up it becomes idolatry.

"When you sit to dine with a ruler, note well what is before you, and put a knife to your throat if you are given to gluttony. Do not crave his delicacies, for that food is deceptive" (Proverbs 23:1-3 NIV). It is sometimes hard to say NO! We find ourselves with others who are celebrating; maybe they

> When we use food for comfort and an emotional pick-up it becomes idolatry.

60

have even prepared something just for us. This is deceptive food! The deception is that we are eating to please man and not God. The devil will be perched on our shoulder telling us that we do not want to hurt their feelings; just one little bite won't hurt. That is how we got into this mess in the first place, just one more bite! Remember, happy is he who does not condemn himself. Obeying what we know is right will satisfy our soul which is much more rewarding than satisfying our taste buds.

I have always found it interesting that Jesus talked about food and doing the will of the Father. The disciples had gone to town for food when Jesus was talking to the woman at the well. When the disciples urged him to eat, he responded, "I have food to eat of which you do not know" (John 4:32). "The disciples said to one another, 'Has anyone brought Him anything to eat?' " (vs. 33). Jesus said to them, "My food is to do the will of Him who sent Me and to finish His work" (vs. 34). He then starts speaking of the fields that are ready for harvest. He is exhorting His disciples to keep their focus. We cannot get consumed with food for the body and forget our purpose. Nothing feeds our spirit like walking in obedience and doing the will of the Father. The will of the Father is to take care of our bodies so we can do the work of the Father. Doing the will of the Father was more important to Jesus than the food He ate. Godly attitudes and character developed in our lives from reading the Word of God will change our behavior.

> Be aware of the scales! They sit there quiet and unassuming, a perfect tool for satan to use to set your mood.

Each pound we lose is evidence of our obedience. Yes, we will sacrifice some things, but obedience is better than sacrifice. There is no comparison to walking with a clear conscious before God. Remember, nothing tastes as good as obedience!

Be aware of the scales! They sit there quiet and unassuming, a perfect tool for satan to use to set your mood. We allow a piece of manmade metal to influence our mind set for the day! If my weight is down, the day is good; if my weight is up, discouragement takes over. Every donut, candy, ice cream, and cookie you have ever seen will be dancing across your mind and want to comfort you. We know we can eat right and not lose weight because there are other things besides the food we eat that can affect our weight.

So use wisdom. I don't get on the scales more than once a week. In the past, I have been addicted to the scales allowing them to show me how I am doing and not depending on my eating habits for the long term goal. My clothes size tells me what I need to know. What joy to put on a dress you haven't been able to wear for several years!

> Our focus must change from weight loss to a healthy lifestyle and walking in obedience to God.

Our focus must change from weight loss to a healthy lifestyle and walking in obedience to God. The Word of God says in Hosea 4:6, "My people are destroyed for lack of knowledge…" This is true in the spirit and in the natural. The problem is we must first want to be taught. I have to confess that I had never studied nutrition. Of course, I'd heard plenty of people talking about good nutrition, but just never studied to show myself approved on the subject. Instead I just continued to believe the lie of the enemy and kept getting fatter.

My focus was on 'weight loss' and there were many diet plans and schemes out there just waiting for me. When I followed one of these plans, I lost weight, but did it stay off? No, because I had not changed my thinking and my purpose for weight loss. I found that the diet industry treats me like I can't think for myself. They make it easy. Some of them prepackage my meals to the right proportion so I don't have to think about what I am eating.

When you buy into this plan they don't tell you it is a life commitment. As soon as you go off the plan, the pounds start rolling on again and you are in for another roller coaster ride because convenience outweighed commitment. We are bombarded today by the views of the world as to our place in society and what brings happiness. There is only one source of power that can stand against the pressure of society, the power of the Holy Spirit. The life of Jesus Christ is the only standard we must follow on this journey through life.

Knowledge brings freedom. Our bodies are fearfully and wonderfully made (Psalm 139:14). "For you were bought at a price; therefore glorify God in your body and in your spirit, which are God's" (1 Corinthians 6:20). Your body is important. For too long as Christians we have placed so much importance on our spiritual condition, which is important, but we have neglected our bodies.

> *"But you are not in the flesh, but in the Spirit,*
> *if indeed the Spirit of God dwells in you. Now*
> *if anyone does not have the Spirit of Christ,*
> *He is not His. And if Christ is in you, the body is*
> *dead because of sin, but the Spirit is life*
> *because of righteousness. But if the Spirit of Him*
> *who raised Jesus from the dead dwells in you,*
> *He who raised Christ from the dead will also*
> *give life to your mortal bodies through His*
> *Spirit who dwells in you" (Romans 8:9-11).*

How amazing this is! The Holy Spirit gives life to our body! We are to glorify God in our bodies. When we get a revelation of the purpose of our bodies, then we will not abuse our bodies with food, drugs, cigarettes, alcohol or any other overindulgence that gratifies the flesh. The body is a vehicle to carry the Holy Spirit and fulfill the great commission in life.

How we care for our bodies is very important. We are to protect the environment of our bodies to guard our heart and mind from the influence of the world. I thank God every day for His mercy in my life. I had carried extra weight for many years and my health has been excellent. I know it is His mercy and I have asked Him to forgive me for neglecting my body.

> One thing I have learned in my Christian walk is that I had to be diligent!

One thing I have learned in my Christian walk is that I had to be diligent! "But without faith it is impossible to please Him, for he who comes to God must believe that He is, and that He is a rewarder of those who diligently seek Him" (Hebrews 11:6). Proverbs 12:27 tells us that diligence is man's precious possession. He is a rewarder of those who diligently seek Him! How and when does He reward us? I asked the Lord once, "What is my reward?" Immediately I heard in my spirit, "revelation knowledge". Revelation knowledge is knowledge that is revealed to you by the Holy Spirit. It is that nugget of truth that reveals the mysteries of the Kingdom of Heaven. When we receive that nugget, faith comes and we please God! "Now faith is the substance of things hoped for, the evidence of things not seen" (Hebrews 11:1).

We must have faith to overcome the ways of the world. "For whatever is born of God (that is you) overcomes the world, and this is the victory that overcomes the world—our faith" (1 John 5:4).

Hope and faith work together. Faith is the substance of things hoped for. When we do things the world's way and our plans fail, we often feel hopeless. There was a woman in the Bible with an issue of blood for 12 years (Mark 5:25-34). She went to many physicians and spent all she had and was no better, but rather grew worse. But one day she heard about Jesus! She reached out and touched the hem of His garment and was immediately healed. Jesus felt the power leave Him and asked who had touched him. The disciples told Him there was a multitude around you and you ask who touched you! But only one had touched Him in faith!

I believe we can learn from this testimony. This woman did not lose hope in the midst of her situation, even when the world gave up on her. Her hope was the driving force that took her to Jesus. Faith is the substance of things hoped for. Hope empowers us to believe. Faith empowers us to receive. Hope perceives, faith receives!

Hope is vital to our faith. Proverbs 13:12 says that "Hope deferred makes the heart sick, but when the desire comes it is a tree of life." What defers our hope? Do you get mad at God when He doesn't answer your prayer when you think He should? Do we get angry and bitter when nothing seems to be working? When we have tried every diet and still have not lost the unwanted pounds do we give up hope? Are we jealous because someone has lost weight and we haven't? Do we constantly compare ourselves with someone else? These are issues of the heart. The Word of God says, "Keep your heart with all diligence, for out of it spring the issues of life" (Proverbs 4:23). When our heart is sick there is no faith. We become self-centered by thinking on the problem and not seeking the Lord for the solution. Our heart is sick and only the Holy Spirit can bring healing as we open our heart to the Lord and ask for His help. Ask the Lord to bring you help. If you don't attend

> It is a ploy of the enemy to keep you alone and try to make you believe you are the only one with this problem and that there is no hope.

church regularly, then start. A great help is to find a Bible Study or support group to help you become accountable. The Lord did not design us to bear our burdens alone. It is a ploy of the enemy to keep you alone and try to make you believe you are the only one with this problem and that there is no hope. There is hope and hope does not disappoint (Romans 5:5).

God has promised to meet all of our needs according to His riches in Glory by Christ Jesus. (Philippians 4:19). This is not an overnight journey, but a life time pursuit. As we learn to trust the Lord, having confidence in Him to meet all our needs, then we will walk in obedience and receive the promise.

"If they obey and serve Him, they shall spend their days in prosperity and their years in pleasures."

(JOB 36:11)

9

Identity: The Secret of Success

> *"But as many as received Him, to them He gave the right to become children of God, to those who believe in His name: who were born, not of blood, nor of the will of the flesh, nor of the will of man, but of God."*

(JOHN 1:12–13)

Most people identify themselves by the roles they play in life. When they do this there is constant confusion and upheaval because our roles in life change. In our life we always play the lead role and it is always opening night. I'm a wife, mother, grandmother, friend, teacher and author, but these roles do not define my identity. My roles change continually, several times a day. I am a child of God. That is my identity and what gives me purpose in my life. When I am confident in my identity, then my roles in life reflect Christ Jesus.

When I accepted Jesus and became a child of God He set my course in life. Now I must learn the rights and privileges I have as a child of God. I had been a slave to sin, and the ways of the world, even if I did not realize it.

Receiving Christ and being born into the family of God gives us a secure relationship. We now qualify for fellowship with God and friendship with Jesus. The relationship is available, but it is up to us to pursue it. It requires honesty. He already knows all our needs, our fears and failures. He wants you to reveal yourself to Him and speak the truth. No hiding from God!

We have a need to be accepted and crave the attention of others telling us they approve. In Him we have been accepted and we are the beloved. Our need for approval is met in Christ Jesus. We are not dependent on our own performance. We no longer fear our failures; we can cultivate the new creation God has allowed us to be in Him.

When we come to Christ most of us are carrying a lot of baggage from the hurts and heartaches we have gathered as we walked through this world. We must learn to take the fertilizer that has been dumped on us and grow roses! We learn early in life to cover-up and hide our insecurities.

> We must learn to take the fertilizer that has been dumped on us and grow roses!

Most people are three in one. The person we think we are, the person we want others to think we are and the one we really are.

We are now on a journey with the help of the Holy Spirit to unwrap ourselves to uncover who we really are. The most important product of your effort is the development of your own character. We live in a false world. We have false teeth, false eye lashes, and false hair. We have push up bras and can shrink wrap our bodies to make them look thinner! Will the real person please stand up!

Now, I really don't have a problem with some of these things. I've always said if the barn needs painted, then paint it! I look pretty much the same as I did 20 years ago; it just takes me a little longer to get there.

It is time we took the mask off and found our real identity, the real person that was created in the image and likeness of God.

When you discover the 'original' you, that God has designed you to be, you will have a well-adjusted, contented, peaceful life no matter what is going on around you. Whatever life has been up to now has shaped and molded us into who we are today. The negative incidents in our past will disable us today if we grant them the power.

> We are now on a journey with the help of the Holy Spirit to unwrap ourselves to uncover who we really are.

We cannot change our past history, but we can allow the Holy Spirit to change the effect of the past on our present. The key to unlocking the past is to get honest and walk in forgiveness. Remember, forgiveness is not about the other person, it is about you. When Christ received me, He forgave my sins. Now I must be willing to forgive others that have sinned against me.

Many people are victims of circumstances. Life is faced with many challenges, but we cannot afford to get bogged down in life with pity parties and unforgiveness. When you study the people in the Bible, you will find that those used the greatest by God were often treated the worst in the world.

Abigail was a victim. Her testimony starts in 1 Samuel 25. She had every excuse to hide herself and feel sorry for what life had given her. Her husband had been chosen for her by her parents. He was a very wealthy man and her parents probably thought they had done well for their daughter. It didn't take Abigail long to figure out that he was a cruel man, an abusive alcoholic.

She was not schooled in the ways of the world, but she had learned much from the dealings of her husband. She did not permit the unfairness of life to squelch her strength in the spirit. When she heard of her husband's wrong doings against David, she quickly took action. Taking supplies to David she met him on the road and faced him with his responsibility to God and Israel. David accepted the courageous woman's provisions and stopped his mission of revenge. Read the testimony and be encouraged in your life as you see how this woman that had been the victim became the wife of the king.

She had every reason to believe she was a loser and to feel sorry for herself. Perhaps there was something wrong with her? God had equipped Abigail to be an overcomer. She had what it took to overcome the injustice against her. She did not question her identity and her purpose in life. Just as Joseph said, the things that had been done to him had been meant for evil, but God had meant it for good. God loves to recycle. He is willing to recycle our past when we give it to Him and allow our unveiling to begin.

> When you are confident in your identity as a child of God you are on the road to success.

Sad to say that even the church has its own set of masks to hide behind. There are many frustrated men and women in church because they have never allowed the Holy Spirit to do an extreme make-over. Instead we hide and fight guilt and rejection and never enjoy the abundant life that Christ died for.

Women feel they must conform, men feel they have to perform, but God tells us to be transformed.

Until we see Jesus face to face, our job is to become the 'real person' created in His image, reflecting that image to the world. We overcome in this world by allowing the Holy Spirit to teach us the ways of the Kingdom and follow Jesus' command to bring Heaven to earth.

When you are confident in your identity as a child of God you are on the road to success. The first temptation that Jesus faced in the wilderness was His identity. "The devil said to Him, if you are the Son of God..." (Luke 4:3). He was trying to cause Jesus to doubt who He was. His power and authority was in His identity, the Son of God.

In the garden the first temptation for Eve was to doubt God's Word; "Has God indeed said..." (Genesis 3:1). Satan constantly uses these same two temptations on us. He knows when we doubt God's word it will cause us to doubt our identity.

When we accept Jesus, we can discover the real person we were created to be in Christ. We now have a solid rock to build our identity upon and cultivate a friendship with Jesus, your best friend! As a child of God we don't have to seek success, it will follow us as we follow Him.

"Don't copy the behavior and customs of this world, but be a new and different person with a fresh newness in all you do and think. Then you will learn from your own experience how His ways will really satisfy you."

(ROMANS 12:2 TLB)

10

Diligence Overcomes Desperation!

"...but diligence is man's precious possession."

(PROVERBS 12:27)

Desperation is a good thing if it turns us toward God. He hears the cry of desperate people.

It seems to be the way of the human race, after all else fails, to turn to God. It is easier to blame God for our failures than to believe God for help. Blaming God takes no effort on our part. To believe God's Word we have to fight against the lies of the enemy, against the powers of darkness and principalities in heavenly places. (Ephesians 6:12). As we have said before, this is a battle and we must be willing to fight for the desires of our heart.

When life is going our way, we tend to forget. We take God's blessings for granted. Psalm 78:40-43 gives us insight into the struggles of the children of Israel to reach the promised land of milk and honey. "How often they provoked Him in the wilderness, and grieved

73

Him in the desert! Yes, again and again they tempted God and limited the Holy One of Israel. They did not remember His power; the day when He redeemed them from the enemy, when He worked His signs in Egypt, and His wonders in the field of Zoan."

I am always amazed when I read this scripture. They limited the Holy One of Israel because they did not remember His power. They saw the Red Sea open and walked through it for their deliverance. I bet as they were walking through the Red Sea with water standing on each side, they said, "I'll never forget this!" They lived every day in the land of miracles with the manna from God. How could they forget? Psalm 103:7 gives us an answer. "He made known His ways to Moses, His acts to the children of Israel." God's acts always point to His ways and His nature. To know the ways of God you must have a personal relationship with Him.

The children of Israel did not want a personal relationship. They told Moses to go up the mountain so he could tell them what He said. (Exodus 20:19). Throughout Deuteronomy, Moses constantly told the people that the real threat to their success was not among the enemy tribes that were in the Promised Land; it was the condition of their hearts.

Because they did not know the ways of God and His nature, they soon forgot about the power of God and His ability to invade and overcome impossibilities. Without the awareness of His presence and understanding His ways, revealed from a personal walk with Him, we will not be able to consistently walk in obedience.

How easy it is to forget God's deliverance during times of trouble. We must remember He is our source of life and has given us everything that pertains to life and godliness (2 Peter 1:3). God will meet you in your wilderness

> Our weakness is where He can prove Himself to be our sufficiency.

when you are desperate enough to cry out. There are over 300 references to the wilderness in the Old and New Testament. Remember, Jesus was led into the wilderness by the Holy Spirit. Jesus went into the wilderness filled with the Holy Spirit and came out in the power of the Holy Spirit (Luke 4). There are always valuable lessons learned in our wilderness experiences.

The children of Israel, for example, wandered 40 years in the wilderness before entering the promised land. Deuteronomy 8:2-6 tells us that God led the children of Israel into the wilderness to test them, to know what was in their hearts. When they came out of Egypt, they came out with a slave mentality. They had to learn the ways of God and how to fight to take and keep the promised land. When we are born again and become a new creation in Christ Jesus, we have to learn the ways of the Kingdom of God and how to fight our enemy.

During their time in the wilderness, God did not abandon them; He met their needs in the wilderness. He protected and guided them by a cloud during the day and fire at night and fed them with manna. God does the same for you and me on our journey of faith as He prepares us for our purpose in life. He takes the time to prune us, purge us and prepare us for our next step of the journey of life.

I believe that we can prolong the journey or shorten the journey by our attitudes and our willingness to surrender. Many people try to have victory without surrender. The children of Israel prolonged their wilderness experience because they limited the Holy One of Israel when they failed to remember.

> Many people try to have victory without surrender.

Their lack of faith, their rebellion and their double-minded ways stopped them from moving forward. They were content with manna when milk and honey were just around the corner! They were fed, but not filled, sustained but not satisfied. Why? They were not desperate enough to cry out for help. They refused to surrender their wills to God. They did not put God first by learning His ways so they would remember His faithfulness and walk in obedience. Three keys to help you overcome—read, remember and obey. James tells us to not be a forgetful hearer of the Word. (James 1:23-25).

Another key to overcoming and entering our promised land is diligence. The definition of diligence is persistent effort, attentive care, and heedfulness. Proverbs 12:27 says that diligence is man's precious possession. The Holy Spirit in us will not allow us to give up! Remember we are not alone in this battle; we have a helper, the Holy Spirit, to help us in our time of need. Hebrews 11:6 says, "But without faith it is impossible to please Him, for he who comes to God must believe that He is, and that He is a rewarder of those who diligently seek Him."

> There is a reward for your diligence. The Holy Spirit is going to open the eyes of your understanding and lead you into all truth and the truth will set you free.

There is a reward for your diligence. The Holy Spirit is going to open the eyes of your understanding and lead you into all truth and the truth will set you free. We must know the truth and live in truth. The source of our truth is the Word of God. Jesus said, "I am the way, the truth, and the life" (John 14:6). Your diligence in the Word of God will overcome your desperation. Life is a gift to enjoy, not a problem to solve. Most people are always trying to solve the problem, instead of resting in the Lord and allowing Him to turn all things for good. Hebrews 11:6 says, without faith it is impossible to please Him. I have heard many sermons, preached a few myself, and have given much thought to the subject of faith. Faith is not something we are striving for, it is a lifestyle of rest and trust. When I first began my faith walk, I thought I had to build my faith to move the mountain. This brings bondage, not rest. I finally figured out that I had to build my faith in God; He was the one who moved the mountain! It was not about me, it was all about Him!

We can only trust the Lord as we build a relationship with Him. Faith is knowing His Word and trusting Him to be faithful to His Word. Faith is having the confidence to ask. "Now this is the confidence that we have in Him, that if we ask anything according to His will, He hears us. And if we know that He hears us, whatever we ask, we know that we have the petitions that we have asked of Him" (1 John 5:14-15). Faith grows in rest. Faith grows as we study and learn who He is and learn His ways.

One of the best ways to learn about God is to study the lives of the men and women in the Bible. Romans 15:4 tells us, "For whatever things were written before were written for our learning, that we through the patience and comfort of the Scripture might have hope." There is nothing new under the sun. The challenges that faced these men and women are the same as the ones we face today. As we see how God delivered those that walked before us and how He brought redemption to us, we begin to understand His love toward us. When we accept His love, faith begins to work in our heart.

> When we accept His love, faith begins to work in our heart.

Faith functions in peace. We must be diligent to fight for peace! How do we do that? I'm glad you asked. "Be anxious for nothing, but in everything by prayer and supplication, with thanksgiving, let your requests be made known to God; and the peace of God, which surpasses all understanding, will guard your hearts and minds through Christ Jesus" (Phil. 4:6-7). I love this, it "surpasses all understanding!" I love walking in that peace where there is nothing that the enemy can throw at you to stop you. All the ugly thoughts just bounce off your helmet of salvation and you stick the sword of the Spirit right in the gut of the enemy and he has to bow his knee.

You have to let your request be made known to God. YOU have to ASK! I don't know how this all works, but I do know my responsibility. I must be diligent in seeking understanding of the mysteries of the Kingdom of heaven (Matthew 13:11) by abiding in the Word (John 15) and out of my heart shall flow rivers of living waters. The secret of asking is abiding. John 15:7 tells us "If you abide in Me, and My words abide in you, you will ask what you desire and it shall be done for you." You will ask! When your heart is full, out of the abundance of the heart, the mouth will speak! (Matt. 12:34).

> The secret of asking is abiding.

Another key I have learned in my own life is that of being accountable. We must be responsible for our own actions. When we look to others to make up our minds, we are not being accountable for our actions. We are taking ourselves off the hook, so if it doesn't work we can blame someone or something else. The decision has to be your own, but there are many support groups available to help you overcome your problem whether it is emotional, physical or spiritual.

We are all created uniquely and what works for one person might not work for another. A diet by definition is described as "the usual or regular foods a person eats most frequently." Everyone is on a diet! Food is not the problem; it is the choices that we make. Our goal in life should be this—"that I may know Him and the power of His resurrection" (Philippians 3:10). When we keep our focus on Him, everything else falls into place.

You must be diligent because the devil, your enemy, walks about like a roaring lion, seeking whom he may devour (1Peter 5:8). The principles in this book apply to our lives in any area that is not surrendered to

> When we keep our focus on Him, everything else falls into place.

the Lord, not just a weight problem. We must plan by the principles, but live in His presence. It is in the presence of the Lord that we hear His voice and feel His pleasure.

Food is not the problem; it is the choices that we make.

To be the best that we can, we must accept our responsibility, look at the options and take action! Success is not a destination; it's a journey of right choices!

Enjoy the journey, the rewards are great and the eating is good!

"...To him who overcomes I will give to eat from the tree of life, which is in the midst of the Paradise of God."

(REVELATION 2:7)

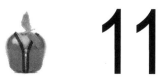

11

One More Word

> "...*for the joy of the Lord is your strength.*"
>
> **(NEHEMIAH 8:10)**

On this journey I have gained much more than I have lost. If my heart doesn't change, it doesn't matter what I do to change my body. If my joy doesn't come from within, then it will not last.

I have found that happy hour is every hour for the child of God. I don't have to wait until 5 pm to go to some bar to get happy!

I have come to accept myself exactly as God created me. I refuse to compare myself with anyone. I was created in His image and likeness and have accepted my responsibility to take care of myself. I will no longer make excuses and blame others for my body shape! God deliberately created me as a unique individual. Enjoy your uniqueness and stop comparing yourself to a friend or family member.

We all lose differently. I have never understood why it seems that men lose weight so easily. I remember my father would say, "I need to lose a few pounds," and he would stop eating popcorn and the weight was gone! I look at popcorn and my hips begin to expand.

We all have different metabolisms. Some of us seem to be in high gear and others just chug along. We must stop worrying what other people think. When you see others eating whatever they want and never seem to gain, remember the food is doing just as much damage to their arteries as it did to yours, no matter what size they are. When we reach the point where we stop comparing ourselves with others and accept our uniqueness as a person created in His image, then we have made progress.

> The Promise Land is not a destination, but a lifestyle!

The Promised Land is not a destination, but a lifestyle. I've been through the Red Sea with the enemy on my tail. I have marched through the desert facing the dangers and traps of the enemy. I've spent time at the bitter waters and crossed the Jordan River and thank God for all I have learned and the sixty pounds I have lost.

As always we look to Jesus, the author and finisher of our faith. "Therefore we also, since we are surrounded by so great a cloud of witnesses, let us lay aside every weight, and the sin which so easily ensnares us, and let us run with endurance the race that is set before us. Looking unto Jesus, the author and finisher of our faith, who for the joy that was set before Him endured the cross, despising the shame, and has sat down at the right hand of the throne of God" (Hebrews 12:1-2).

> Food is not a sin, but when it has control over us it becomes a weight that easily ensnares us.

Lay aside every weight (no pun intended!). A weight is that which brings bondage in your life which keeps you from enjoying the joy of the Lord. Food is not a sin, but when it has control over us it becomes a weight that easily ensnares us.

Let us run with endurance the race that is set before us because we can see beyond the natural world we live in and taste the joy of accomplishing His purpose in our lives.

During a very dark hour in his own life Paul wrote to the Philippian Church. The central theme is: only in Christ is real unity and joy possible. Paul exhorts the church to "stand fast…be of the same mind…rejoice in the Lord always…but in everything by prayer and supplication, with thanksgiving, let your requests be made known…and the peace of God, which surpasses all understanding, will guard your hearts and minds through Christ Jesus" (4:1,2,4,6,7). No matter where you are in your journey, keep these verses in your heart. No matter what the circumstances in your life are, it is the joy of the Lord that will take you through the dark times and bring victory.

I continue the race that is set before me. Am I wearing a size 2? No, and I never will. I am happy and healthy and that is the goal. I have lost 65 pounds and according to the world's standard could lose another 20. I will continue to eat right and exercise. Exercise is a subject that wasn't covered in this book and I have never enjoyed it. But when I heard the words— "walk on purpose for His purpose," I was obedient. One thing I do enjoy is being in the water, so I take a water aerobics class three days a week and walk 3 days a week.

> Life is tough, even with Jesus on board, but it is impossible without him.

Life is tough, even with Jesus on board, but it is impossible without him. Walking in the light while living in a dark world is not an easy assignment. It is a daily walk. Too many of us are living in regrets of the past or in fantasies for the future. We can always start next Monday. No, today is the day of salvation!

I haven't arrived yet, but I have left and God isn't finished with me! "But none of these things move me; nor do I count my life dear to myself, so that I may finish my race with joy, and the ministry which I received from the Lord Jesus, to testify to the gospel of the grace of God" (Acts 20:24).

*We have
tasted and seen
that
the Lord is good!*

The Battle Plan

"...There is a natural body, and there is a spiritual body."

(1CORINTHIANS 15:44)

We need to take care of both!

Spiritual Body

- **Pray** for wisdom and a divine strategy for you. You are unique and God has a plan just for you. Prayer is your power source. Remember we were told to ask and receive that our joy might be full. (John 16:24)
- **Ask** the Lord for a "word" spoken to your heart— a word from the Lord gives you the faith to overcome the battle.
- **Cultivate** a lifestyle of worship and thanksgiving.
- **Build** yourself up praying in the Holy Spirit. Ask the Holy Spirit for revelation knowledge. (Jude 20)
- **Fasting** is a gateway to the supernatural. Ask the Holy Spirit to lead you in this.
- **Purpose** in your heart to have a quiet time every day, even if it is 10 minutes.

- **Accountability**—find a support group, a Bible Study or a friend to share your challenges and victories. Keep a success journal. Include prayer request and answers, and scriptures that encourage you.
- **Meditate** Psalm 139:13-16 and 1 Corinthians 6:19-20. *When you have a revelation of the purpose of your body you will not abuse it.* The purpose of your body is to carry the message of the Lord Jesus Christ and a dwelling place for the Holy Spirit.

Natural Body

- **Learn:** Settle in your heart a food plan for yourself. Study nutrition and how it affects the body and what causes the food cravings we have. Knowledge brings freedom. Through knowledge you gain wisdom to make wise choices. There are many good websites that help you learn about food and its nutritional value.
- **Plan:** Preparation and planning is a way to escape those run-a-way thoughts. You know what you are eating and you won't be tempted to grab something to stop the craving and hunger pangs. Look for new recipes that will fit your lifestyle.
- **Track:** Write down what you eat every day. You will not have to do this forever. In the beginning it helps you understand what food helps you lose weight. It is a tool to keep you on the right track.
- **Commitment:** Changing your lifestyle and eating habits requires commitment, hard work and dedication. Be committed to keeping yourself healthy and happy. This is not a "temporary fix," but a permanent change in eating habits that will give you the long happy life that you are promised by God!

This is a life time commitment to walk in freedom from bondage and enjoy the life that has been given to you. Don't be in a hurry, rest and relax in this journey called life.

The devil wants you fat, it is part of his plan to kill, steal and destroy your happiness and stop you from the plans and purposes that God has for your life.

You are smarter than the devil and you have an advantage over the world, you have a helper, the Holy Spirit. Keep your focus on your spiritual body and the natural will follow.

"But seek first the Kingdom of God and His righteousness, and all these things shall be added to you."

(MATTHEWS 6:33)

Keep in touch. Visit the website: www.whydiets.com and let us hear your success testimonies.

Schedule a "Why Weight" Seminar and experience the joy and power of the Holy Spirit as we come together in one spirit to defeat our enemy!

Points to Ponder

Chapter 1

He spoke and I Was Strengthened

God speaks today. To follow Him we must hear His voice. (John 10:4)

Faith comes from hearing His voice.
(Romans 10:17)

Reading and meditating the Word of God gives us the capacity to hear the voice of God. The Holy Spirit reveals the Word of God to us and leads us as we walk the runway of life.

Chapter 2

A Lack of Perception Leads to Deception

The only weapon the serpent has is deception and your weapon is the Word of God hidden in your heart, asking the Holy Spirit to reveal that Word to you. He will bring to your remembrance the Word that you need for deliverance.

The serpent deceived Eve by causing her to question God's Word. "Has God indeed said…" (Genesis 3:1)

Joyce Tilney

Hide the Word of God in your heart that you will not sin against God. (Psalm 119:11)

Chapter 3

It's an Inside Job!

We must change on the inside before we will change on the outside. Change on the inside comes from renewing our mind with the Word of God.

The difference we make with our lives is contingent on the difference we allow God to make in our lives.

Chapter 4

Created in His Image

We are created in His image and His likeness. We are a spirit, we have a soul and live in a body. Study spirit, soul and body continually so you grow in your understanding of how you were created to function in this world as a child of God.
This is a lifetime experience.

Your spirit is king, your soul a servant and your body a slave. Our bodies will follow our mind set. The body does not think or make decisions. It is a slave to our soul and our soul needs to be directed by our spirit. When we get a revelation of the purpose of our body, we will not abuse it!

Chapter 5

The Battle of The Bulge

In every battle you face, you need to know your enemy and how he operates. The mind is the battlefield. Satan is clever, his suggestions are so subtle that he can take thoughts that we know are wrong and make them appear to be right.

We must take the weapons of our warfare and cast down every thought that is against the Word of God. To be able to do that, we must know the Word of God.

Chapter 6

You've Been Around This Mountain Long Enough!

It is easier to live in a rut than to break a habit. As you go around your mountain you feel comfortable, you see your old friends and you know what to expect.

It starts with making the decision that I will walk in obedience and that I will ask the Holy Spirit to help me. Only by the power of the Holy Spirit that is within you can you break the yoke of bondage that has you snared.

Chapter 7

Fasting, The Weapon of Choice

Fasting is not just going without food for a certain time— that is dieting. Biblical fasting is refraining from food for a spiritual purpose.

Fasting is a choice. Fasting is a gateway to the supernatural— breaking out of the routine to draw near to God. When you study the Word of God you will see in the Old and New Testament, fasting was a part of an ongoing lifestyle.

Living a fasted lifestyle keeps you sensitive and alert to the deception of the enemy. Most people fast in a crisis. If you live a lifestyle of prayer and fasting you might avoid a few of the crisis in your life, as you become sensitive and alert to the warnings in your spirit.

If Jesus could do everything He was sent to do without fasting, why would He fast? He knew there was supernatural strength that could only be released by fasting. When you fast, your mind becomes uncluttered by the things of this world and your spirit becomes more sensitive to the things of God.

Chapter 8

Nothing Tastes As Good As Obedience

As you walk in obedience, the joy and peace that comes is better than the weight loss! The weight loss is just an added benefit.

Obedience is better than sacrifice (1 Samuel 15:22). Each pound we lose is evidence of our obedience. Yes, there will be some sacrifices— our taste buds will scream and our stomachs will growl, but what do they know? Remember, they got you into trouble in the first place.

Chapter 9

Identity, The Secret of Success

Your confidence in life comes from knowing your identity. Most people think of their role in life as their identity. Roles change, identity does not. You are a child of God and you have the right to understand and know the mysteries of the Kingdom of Heaven.

When you are confident in your identity as a child of God you are on the road to success. The first temptation that Jesus faced in the wilderness was His identity. "The devil said to Him, 'if you are the Son of God...' (Luke 4:3). He was trying to cause Jesus to doubt who He was because His strength was in His identity, the Son of God.

In the garden the first temptation for Eve was to doubt God's Word; "Has God indeed said..." (Genesis 3:1). Satan constantly uses these same two temptations on us. He knows when we doubt God's word it will cause us to doubt our identity.

Chapter 10

Diligence Overcomes Desperation!

Desperation is a powerful force. Desperation is a good thing if it turns your heart to the Lord. So often we must become desperate before we seek the Lord for help.

Overcoming desperation comes from diligence. God blesses diligence. (Hebrews 11:6)

Chapter 11

One More Word

The joy of the Lord is your strength! (Neh. 8:10). No matter what is going on in this world, you are on your way to heaven. (As long as you have received Jesus as your savior).

I love the words of Jesus as He was preparing the disciples for His departure. "These things I have spoken to you, that My joy may remain in you and that your joy may be full."
(John 15:11).

"...Ask, and you will receive, that your joy may be full."
(John 16:24).

Joy is a fruit of the spirit. (Galatians 5:22) Fruit is grown as we learn to trust the Lord.

Above all else....

Remember, you are not alone in this battle, or any battle in your life! You have a helper, the Holy Spirit.

Keep yourself cleansed by the washing of the water of the Word (Ephesians 5:26).

Meditate on The Word day and night and YOU will make your way prosperous as you walk the runway of life (Joshua 1:8).

Always have a heart of thanksgiving that He is with you and in the midst of every battle in life!

"But now, thus says the Lord, who created you, O Jacob, and He who formed you, O Israel; Fear not, for I have redeemed you; I have called you by your name; YOU are mine" (Isaiah 43:1).

Jacob's name was changed to Israel (Genesis 32:28). Jacob was created and Israel was formed through the trials of life. He had struggled with God and with men and he prevailed!

You too will prevail as you keep your eyes on Jesus, the author and finisher of your faith.

God loves you, you are the apple of His eye!

Words for the walk, one step at a time, looking beyond past failure and into a successful future!

"Man shall not live by bread alone, but by every word that proceeds from the mouth of God" (Matthew 4:4).

"Blessed are those who hunger and thirst for righteousness, for they shall be filled" (Matthew 5:6).

"I have not departed from the commandments of His lips; I have treasured the words of His mouth more than my necessary food" (Job 23:12).

"They willfully put God to the test by demanding the food they craved" (Psalm 78:18 NIV).

"My food is to do the will of Him who sent Me, and to finish His work" (John 4:34).

"Or do you not know that your body is the temple of the Holy Spirit, who is in you, whom you have from God, and you are not your own? For you were bought at a price; therefore glorify God in your body and in your spirit, which are God's" (1 Corinthian 6:19-20).

"Do not join those who drink too much wine or gorge themselves on meat, for drunkards and gluttons become poor, and drowsiness clothes them in rags" (Proverbs 23:20-21 NIV).

"For He satisfies the longing soul, and fills the hungry soul with goodness" (Psalm 107:9).

"Finally, brethren, whatever things are true, whatever things are noble, whatever things are just, whatever things are pure, whatever things are lovely, whatever are of good report, if there is any virtue and if there is anything praiseworthy—meditate on these things" (Philippians 4:8).

"May God himself, the God of peace, sanctify you through and through. May your whole spirit, soul and body be kept blameless at the coming of our Lord Jesus Christ" (1 Thessalonians 5:23 NIV).

"All things are lawful for me, but all things are not helpful. All things are lawful for me, but I will not be brought under the power of any" (1 Corinthians 6:12).

"Do you not know that to whom you present yourselves slaves to obey, you are that one's slaves whom you obey, whether of sin leading to death, or of obedience leading to righteousness?" (Romans 6:16).

"whose end is destruction, whose god is their belly, and whose glory is in their shame—who set their mind on earthly things" (Philippians 3:19).

"These things I have spoken to you while being present with you. But the Helper, the Holy Spirit, whom the Father will send in My name, He will teach you all things, and bring to your remembrance all things that I said to you" (John 14:25-26).

"These things I have spoken to you, that you should not be made to stumble" (John 16:1).

"...and these things I speak in the world, that they may have My joy fulfilled in themselves" (John 17:13).

"These things I have spoken to you, that in Me you may have peace. In the world you will have tribulation; but be of good cheer, I have overcome the world" (John 16:33).

"Nevertheless I tell you the truth, it is to your advantage that I go away; for if I do not go away, the Helper will not come to you; but if I depart, I will send Him to you" (John 16:7). You have an advantage over the world! You have a helper, the Holy Spirit.

"To the praise of the glory of His grace, by which He made us accepted in the Beloved" (Ephesians 1:6).

Spirit Food for the Spirit Man

"Restore to me the joy of your salvation and grant me a willing spirit, to sustain me" (Psalm 51:12 NIV).

"Watch and pray so that you will not fall into temptation. The spirit is willing, but the body is weak" (Matthew 26:41 NIV).

"But because my servant Caleb has a different spirit and follows me wholeheartedly, I will bring him into the land he went to, and his descendants will inherit it" (Numbers 14:24 NIV).

"You gave me life and showed me kindness, and in your providence watched over my spirit" (Job 10:12 NIV).

"Into your hands I commit my spirit; redeem me, O Lord, the God of truth" (Psalm 31:5 NIV).

"The tongue that brings healing is a tree of life, but a deceitful tongue crushes the spirit" (Proverbs 15:4 NIV).

"A happy heart makes the face cheerful, but heartache crushes the spirit" (Proverbs 15:13 NIV).

"Create in me a pure heart, O God, and renew a steadfast spirit within me" (Psalm 51:10 NIV).

"'Has not my hand made all these things, and so they came into being? 'declares the Lord. 'This is the one I esteem: he who is humble and contrite in spirit, and trembles at my word'" (Isaiah 66:2 NIV).

"He who has knowledge spares his words, and a man of understanding is of a calm spirit" (Proverbs 17:27).

"The lamp of the Lord searches the spirit of a man; it searches out his inmost being" (Proverbs 20:27 NIV).

"All the ways of a man are pure in his own eyes, but the Lord weighs the spirits" (Proverbs 16:2).

"He who is slow to anger is better than the mighty, and he who rules his spirit than he who takes a city" (Proverbs 16:32).

"But if Christ is in you, your body is dead because of sin, yet your spirit is alive because of righteousness" (Romans 8:10 NIV).

"So it is written: The first Adam became a living being; the last Adam, a life-giving spirit" (1 Corinthians 15:45 NIV).

"And be renewed in the spirit of your mind" (Ephesians 4:23).

"For God did not give a spirit of timidity, but a spirit of power, of love and of self-discipline" (2 Timothy 1:7 NIV).

"Instead, it should be that of your inner self (spirit), the unfading beauty of a gentle and quiet spirit, which is of great worth in God's sight" (1 Peter 3:4 NIV).

"I have heard the rebuke that reproaches me, and the spirit of my understanding causes me to answer" (Job 20:3).

"For I am full of words, and the spirit within me compels me" (Job 32:18 NIV).

"A man's spirit sustains him in sickness, but a crushed spirit who can bear?" (Proverbs 18:14 NIV).

"…My soul glorifies the Lord and my spirit rejoices in God my Savior" (Luke 1:46b–47 NIV).

"For God is my witness, whom I serve with my spirit in the gospel of his Son, that without ceasing I make mention of you always in my prayers" (Romans 1:9).

"For who among men knows the thoughts of man except the man's spirit within him? In the same way no one knows the thoughts of God except the Spirit of God" (1 Corinthians 2:11 NIV).

"The Lord be with your spirit. Grace be with you" (2 Timothy 4:22 NIV).

"The grace of the Lord Jesus Christ be with your spirit" (Philemon 25 NIV).

Soul Food for the Soul

"My soul yearns for you in the night; in the morning my spirit longs for you. When your judgments come upon the earth, the people of the world learn righteousness" (Isaiah 26:9 NIV).

"He restores my soul. He guides me in paths of righteousness for his name's sake" (Psalm 23:3 NIV).

"As the deer pants for streams of water, so my soul pants for you, O God" (Psalm 42:1 NIV).

"The law of the Lord is perfect, converting the soul; the testimony of the Lord is sure, making wise the simple" (Psalm 19:7).

"And do not fear those who kill the body but cannot kill the soul. But rather fear Him who is able to destroy both soul and body in hell" (Matthew 10:28).

"Beloved, I pray that you may prosper in all things and be in health just as your soul prospers" (3 John 2).

Health Food for the Body

"But I discipline my body and bring it into subjection, lest, when I have preached to others, I myself should become disqualified" (1 Corinthians 9:27).

"Therefore I say to you, do not worry about your life, what you will eat or what you will drink; not about your body, what you will put on. Is not life more than food and the body more than clothing?" (Matthews 6:25).

"Or do you not know that your body is the temple of the Holy Spirit who is in you, whom you have from God, and you are not your own?" (1 Corinthian 6:19).

"For as the body without the spirit is dead, so faith without works is dead also" (James 2:26).

"It is sown a natural body, it is raised a spiritual body. There is a natural body, and there is a spiritual body" (1 Corinthians 15:44).

"I beseech you therefore brethren, by the mercies of God, that you present your bodies a living sacrifice, holy, acceptable to God, which is your reasonable service" (Romans 12:1).

Recommended Reading

Spirit, Soul & Body: United in Oneness with God
Lester Sumrall

The Supernatural Power of a Transformed Mind
Bill Johnson

Hosting The Presence: Unveiling Heaven's Agenda
Bill Johnson

Fasting
Jentezen Franklin

The Power of Fasting: 21 Days That Can Change Your Life
Marilyn Hickey

The Daniel Fast
Susan Gregory

If you have never accepted the love of God, now is the time.

God loves you and wants to be connected to you.

Sin separates people from God.

Jesus died for your sins.

"If you confess with your mouth Jesus as Lord, and believe in your heart that God raised Him from the dead, you shall be saved" (Romans 10:9).

You can receive Jesus, enter His Kingdom, and begin your journey of knowing God's love by praying this prayer:

Heavenly Father, I repent of my sins and ask Jesus to come into my heart. I believe you died for my sins and you were raised from the dead. Fill me with your Holy Spirit. Thank you for my salvation. Amen

This is the beginning of a new life. You are now a child of God!

"He came to His own, and His own did not receive Him. But as many as received Him to them He gave the right to become children of God, to those who believe in His name. who were born, not of blood nor of the will of the flesh, nor of the will of man, but of God" (John 1:11-13).

You have received Jesus, now you are a child of God. No matter what the circumstances of your natural birth, you are accepted and you are the beloved!

About the Author

Joyce Tilney, Founder of Women of God Ministries, is a wife, mother and grandmother. Through her practical teaching and humor, women's lives are changed as they understand their role and identity as a woman of God.

Her open and candid teaching style shares personal experiences that impart hope and encouragement for your daily walk as you face the trials of life. She confronts the daily challenges of attitudes— bitterness, worries, jealousy and rejection—issues that stop us from walking in the peace and joy the Lord has promised.

Joyce and her husband Bill lived and ministered in Scotland for 11 years. During this time they pioneered two churches and she began Women of God Ministries. Traveling throughout Europe and Asia she knows and understands that the heart of a woman does not change from culture to culture or century to century.

Joyce teaches in seminars and conference for women as well as traveling with her husband, Bill, team teaching from their rich experience in ministry, family life and marriage.

At this time they live near Philadelphia, Pennsylvania.

Women of God Ministries

Teaching women today from women of yesterday

"For whatever things were written before were written for our learning, that we through the patience and comfort of the Scriptures might have hope."

(ROMANS 15:4)

What better way to build your faith than to study from the women that have walked before us! They are remarkable people with real feelings and real struggles! The heart of a woman does not change from culture to culture or from century to century. Women's needs are the same throughout the ages. They need to belong, to love and be loved, find their identity, develop their gifts and juggle their responsibilities.

- Sarah told her husband what to do, then got mad at him because he did it!
- Eve had everything a woman could want, but was not content.

- Leah, was betrayed by her father, rejected by her husband and hated by her sister, but learned to walk through the trials of life to a place of honor.
- Rebekah received a word from the Lord regarding the birth of her sons, but felt she had to help God fulfill the promise!

Can you relate to these women? Real women facing real problems! Some walked with God, some didn't. We can learn from both.

We are bombarded today by the views of the world as to who a woman is to be and her place in society.

There is only one source of power that can stand against the pressure of society, the power of the Holy Spirit. The life of Jesus Christ is the only standard we must follow on this journey we call life.

True womanhood is not measured by the world's praises or man's attention. Womanhood is measured by a woman's own character developed from the Word of God.

Visit Women of God Ministries website, www.wogministries.com, and share in the blog community as we learn together to be the women God created us to be! Be encouraged in your faith as we share those extraordinary moments with God.

Joyce is available for teaching in your Bible Studies, Seminars and Conferences. Her teaching/prophetic insight imparts life changing revelation that will change your life.

Life is full of pain, but misery is optional for

THE CHILD OF GOD!

Women of God Ministries

Recommended by Men of God

Dick Mills
Dick Mills Ministries

Psalms 68:11 in the Latin vulgate reads, "The Lord gave the Word of deliverance and the female evangelists who proclaimed it were a mighty host."

This verse is very applicable to Joyce Tilney and the anointed ladies making up the Women of God Ministries.

Betty and I have known Bill and Joyce Tilney and have been heart warmed by the work of grace in their lives. It's truly awesome to watch at close range the character development and the spiritual gifting and abilities God has given them both.

Joyce was given by the Lord a vision, a calling and an enablement to teach women the ways of the Lord. She has wisely followed the Lord in a very straight forward and disciplined walk. Her ministry is not a humanly structured program with a fleshly agenda on a calculated plan for building her empire. She is led by the Spirit, moving in the Spirit and anointed by the Spirit to impact women's lives.

One heartwarming facet of the Women of God is how easily her group fits in with all churches and denominations. She is equally at home with all church groups. Another facet that has impressed me is Joyce Tilney's ability to work with all Women's Groups that have invited her. She gets invitations from many Women's organizations all over the world. She fits in easily with these groups because she is not clannish, doesn't have any feelings of elitism or exclusivity or territorial control.

I predict that this group and its sensitive and wise leadership will have a ripple effect that will reach to the ends of the earth to the end of the Church Age.

Edwin Louis Cole

Christian Men's Network

Bill and Joyce Tilney are true friends, and their ministry over the years has matured and now grown to international proportions. Biblically based and Christ centered, they present divine truth to be lived in practical life. Her Women of God conferences are excellent with lasting results. Bill and Joyce are two of God's choice servants and I recommend them without reservation.

Billy Joe Daughtery

Victory Christian Center, Tulsa, OK.

Joyce Tilney is leading a special movement, Women of God Ministries. She was a faithful worker for Victory Christian Center when she and her husband lived in Tulsa, Oklahoma, USA. We rejoice for this hour that women are rising up to the works and spreading the Word of our Lord Jesus Christ.

Robert Garrett, Jr.
Praise Fellowship Church

Joyce is a tremendous role model to women in demonstrating the character of Christ as a woman, wife and mother. She also demonstrates the power of God in ministry as she focuses on women's needs, yet not to the exclusion of men. A wholesomeness and balance is evident in what she accomplishes for the Kingdom of God. Women of God Ministries is not only a fitting title, but a refreshing identity of women and men everywhere. It is an honor and blessing to recommend Joyce Tilney to the Body of Christ.

Schedule a "Why Weight" Seminar in Your Area.

Learn to:

- Hear His Voice.
- Walk in the Spirit.
- Break the cycle of bondage.
- Experience the power of joy.

Joyce has spent years in the struggle of weight issues. This book is enlightening and helps you realize you can put down the shame, anger, resentment and struggle of weight issues.

You do not have to be held captive in your body! By the power of the Word of God and the help of the Holy Spirit you can break the bondage and walk in freedom from the "weightier issues of life."

The purpose of the book is to "whet your appetite"
with the Word of God.
The purpose of a seminar is to establish you in the truth.

Contact Information:

Women of God Ministries, Inc.
PO Box 43, Brandamore, PA 19316
joycetilney@yahoo.com
www.whydiets.com
www.wogministries.com